Stars of the Meadow

Stars of the Meadow

Exploring Medicinal Herbs as Flower Essences

David Dalton

Lindisfarne Books

Credits

The illustrations were done by Sharon Di Giovanni, an artist and nature lover who lives in Northern Maine with her family. She has been passionate about sketching plants since she was a small child.

The repertory section was researched and compiled by Claudia Keel, an herbalist, flower essence practitioner, and artist who teaches in New York City. She conducts workshops in public schools and community gardens about how to create imaginative connections to the natural world.

© David Dalton 2006, 2013

Published by Lindisfarne Books
An imprint of Anthroposophic Press/SteinerBooks
610 Main Street, Great Barrington, Massachusetts 01230
www.steinerbooks.org

Library of Congress Cataloging-in-Publication Data is available.

ISBN: 978-1-58420-035-2

Contents

Foreword

SEVERAL YEARS AGO, when organizing the first Healing with Flowers Conference here in the Northeast, I contacted Patricia Kaminski, the co-director of the Flower Essence Society who immediately suggested that we invite David Dalton to teach at our gathering. Little did we realize how David's teaching would bring us into a deeper intimacy and profound understanding of the power and healing, not only of the flowers in our gardens and wild places, but also of our own personal natures.

David's long and patient years of quietly working with the plants referenced in *Stars of the Meadow* have developed into a remarkable work in progress. What you hold in your hands in the accumulation of much time, devotion, impeccable honesty and the clear light of David's connection and love of the natural world.

The plants he presents in this volume have been used medicinally by past and present herbalists. As a practicing herbalist, it has been my pleasure to extend the application of these healing plants in their individual flower essences when working with people and animals. I am especially grateful for the way David has moved beyond descriptions and indications to more fully develop the true character of each essence and the personality traits of those who could benefit from each of these "stars."

David writes from his rich experience as a therapist and flower essence practitioner in presenting each flower portrait with clarity and fullness. He generously offers the reader the opportunity to develop a relationship with the flowers and use them in one's personal and clinical healing practice. This is an outstanding resource for anyone interested in learning more about the flowers that grace the Northeast fields and woods.

As the "stars" illuminate our paths, so David shines a light before us as a guide and reminder of the beauty, power and healing of the flowers in our meadows.

KATE GILDAY, *Woodland Essence, Cold Brook, New York*

To my mother Anna Dalton
who taught me about love and flowers.

Preface

THIS BOOK represents nearly twenty years of research. Although the plants described here have been used for centuries as medicinal herbs, their healing qualities as flower essences are only now beginning to be understood and used to their potential. Understanding energy has been a crucial part of learning how a plant expresses itself as a flower essence. Until recently we did not have the conceptual tools to explore and learn about these remedies. We literally did not know how to explain what we observed happening except in the most general of terms.

We also had no sense of long- and short-term uses of the essences; how they could help those of us who carried imprints of early trauma that had left scars of physical, mental and emotional pain and turmoil in our lives; what might happen if essences were used to accompany long and short-term psychotherapy. Some of these answers we now have.

My research has included hundreds of adults, children and animals who have been volunteers in research studies or clients in my flower essence practice since the mid-1980s. It has been these cases that have formed both the structure and the content of this work. Without so many willing and satisfied participants, I would not have been able to collect observations into patterns; results into a viable conceptual framework.

For the past ten years I have been teaching courses in flower essences. This has opened the research field to include clients and patients of psychotherapists, veterinarians, herbalists, naturopathic physicians, nurses, homeopaths, educators, and many other professional fields that help guide and heal those who are in physical, mental and emotional pain.

Flower essence students and enthusiasts will enjoy this book, since the flower essence world is thirsty for both structure and data. Within this book there are no projections, extrapolations or leaps of faith. There are no guesses, hunches, hopes or intuitions. Everything presented has unfolded in the stories of many brave pioneers who presented themselves and their pain in a spirit of empirical hopefulness which, in time, became seasoned faith.

With great excitement and heartfelt gratitude I share my experience in this field, hoping the day comes soon when the world sees and accepts the magic, the beauty, the power and tremendous potential available in these simple remedies — a power and potential to heal a sick and wounded world.

DAVID DALTON,
Deltas Gardens, New Hampshire

Introduction

OVER THE YEARS, my work with flower essences has gone through a metamorphosis of sorts. My first explorations into their use were very western, scientific and looking back, all wrong. When we ingest something for health — a pill, a tea and herb — we are programmed to be passive and expect results which are usually the absence of some pain we are treating. We have tendencies here in the west to be one-dimensional and myopic, looking only to the areas that we treat for results. Although my approach with the flower remedies was at first along these lines — I wanted to see if they worked — I could not have been further off the mark.

Of course I got results. But often more than I bargained for and in different ways than I expected. Always the results taught me to open my field of inquiry wider, deeper. I remember treating a young girl for a neurological disorder and discovering that immediately after application of the essence (every time), she would cry about her dog who had passed away years before, or a young boy with eczema whose temperament changed dramatically as his rash subsided, or a teenage girl whose confidence blossomed and grades improved as her asthma cleared. These and many other cases forced me to view, not just the essences, but health and healing differently.

There were many clients who claimed not to have experienced *anything* over a treatment period, but agreed that they felt better, more alive, stronger, and that life seemed to be easier for them. This was apt to recur over several treatment periods until the client had to admit that something was indeed happening. To those who did not "notice" anything I developed a standard response, pointing out what *had* changed and generally promising that such luck, if it were luck, was likely to continue.

In the flower essence domain, the mind and emotions meet the body; the internal and the external are part of the same picture. Luck and chance disappear into creation and manifestation, not as a responsibility we have to meet but as an opportunity to change the way we live our lives.

I began to see physical symptoms, less as something in themselves, and more as part of a larger imbalance of the personality itself. Remember, Dr. Bach had observed that his patients followed a remarkable pattern. The same types of personalities developed the same type of physical illnesses. It was this observation that led him to discover the English or Bach flower essences. Seeing the personality as the center of the treatment and the physical symptoms as secondary launched my practice into another whole direction. And to my satisfaction, if not my surprise, physical symptoms would nearly always improve as the personality came into greater balance.

Another shift in my treatment approach came later as I began to observe relationships between a person's past, his or her inner mental-emotional condition and present satisfaction with the external factors in one's life. It became a standard part of my practice to look at the relationship between a person's history, pain in the psyche and how that pain externalized in the person's life. For instance a common type of picture for me to see was a relationship between sexual trauma in the past and pelvic symptoms in the present accompanied by difficulty maintaining relationships in their lives. In this type of expanded paradigm, flower essences excel, bringing imprints of trauma to the surface where they can be worked with and released. This is one way flower essences work.

I began to see that there was an active participation in the essence taking process which would put the client closer to where the healing action was happening. I would instruct the client to take the essence and to be quiet and "listen" inside. In most cases, this would result in an amplified effect of the essence. It is as if the essences work better when there is cooperation from the human psyche. This practice of "listening" has become part of my standard practice with each client and opens another door for them as active participants in their own healing. Most people, when "listening" or tuning in, will feel some physiological change which can be, at times, profound and the beginning of a new type of relationship with flower essences.

When asked how flower essences work, it is difficult to respond because the question from the western mind asks for a western answer. When asked what flower essences are, the same frustration surfaces since there are certain codes and limitations to our descriptions of substances. What is in this? How do you extract it? The answers are complex and require the construction of a system that begins to explain health in an energetic way; that begins to describe material phenomena in a metaphysical way.

There are many ways that flower essences work, but understanding this means developing a point of view that sees energy, or observes the rhythms and patterns of flower essence results in a way that understands and predicts their action. The study of the chakra system alongside of the shapes and colors of the flowers and the observation of the effects of the essences provides a way of understanding flower essences from their own point of view and within the framework of their own language. Stars of the Meadow gives an energetic explanation of the workings of each flower. This adds to the depth of understanding of both the action and the potential of each essence. It is hoped that it provides both an understandable language and a dependable vehicle for flower essence research now and in the future.

The Chakras

There is an energetic counterpart in the human system for every event. Thoughts, feelings, actions—choices in both the conscious mind and the subconscious—are all represented in energy codes that we can refer to as *vibrations*. Most of the information we have gathered to date on the human energy system is not functional—that is, it does not completely explain the interworkings of the system—what happens when the person is under stress or threat; what happens when there is peace and happiness. The use of colors to represent chakras is only partially true. What we are doing in describing the energy system is attempting to use a language of the physical eyes to explain phenomena that are metaphysical.

Beyond the physical body, the language is *vibration*. There is high, low, dense, ethereal. There are also qualities of the vibration that can be described using the elements. A fiery vibration can be represented with an intense fiery color, etc. Color is a satisfactory language as long as one understands it is a metaphor we are using to describe a quality of energy.

Flowers essences are a language of *vibration*. They have color which essentially helps us to understand and code the vibrations, and most importantly, begin to relate the vibration of the flower to the energy system. Flower essence practitioners and researchers are on the forefront of understanding how the energy system works through investigation of how the personality responds to the vibration of the flower essence itself. Over time the vibration, color, complexity and functionality of the energy system, all reveal themselves through the key of the codes of the plants. The colors, textures, etc., show themselves to be teachers of the energy system by how they affect it.

All lilies, for instance, seem to influence the second chakra directly, while the third chakra is the domain for daisies and the fourth for roses. What happens to these chakras with the intervention of a flower essence, however, is anything but simple. One lily, for instance may bring sexual trauma in the second chakra to the surface, while another may help resolve issues with one's parents. How this happens can be seen in how the essence changes the energetic balance contained in the chakras.

The following is a brief essay on the first three chakras and flower essences. It offers the beginnings of a language that flower essence students may use to explain the depth and complexity of what flower essences are and how they work. It will help with the understanding of each of the essences described in this book, and help serve as a basis for understanding the actions of many other flowers not described here.

CHAKRAS ONE, TWO AND THREE

Chakras are the primary organs of the human energy system. They might be called gateways, portals or centers where energy is collected and distributed throughout the system. Chakras can also be seen as houses or dwelling places for *soul* energy or the individuality of the person as he or she comes into incarnation. This energy moves throughout the system giving life, vitality and consciousness to the individual, physically, mentally, emotionally and spiritually.

The information given here has been developed to assist the flower essence student in understanding, diagnosing and treating imbalances in the system. Flower essences are plant energy. Understanding the structure, function and organization of the human energy system is an ideal way to learn about the use of flower essences.

There are seven basic chakras or centers. Each one performs a different function. Each has a different location. Each has a different configuration or level of health from individual to individual. Each system, however different, has some basic operational truths in common.

They hold energy.

They distribute energy throughout the physical body.

They are dwelling places for soul energy.

Soul energy has a very high vibration.

They are also dwelling places for trauma.

Trauma has a very low vibration.

Soul energy cannot occupy an area of a center which contains trauma.

The higher the vibration of a chakra, the healthier that part of the system will be.

Chakras contain a template of our history. Each few years of our lives is held in a membrane or layer of a chakra. Each membrane has a level of health or vibration. The combined vibration of each layer gives a chakra its "spin" or net energy, which determines a major aspect of its health.

A traumatic event or traumatic period of life will result in a generally darker, lower vibration, which in turn will result in a vulnerability in health in the areas of the physical related to the specific chakras which are influenced. This will become clearer when we talk about the chakras individually.

The goal of flower essence treatment is to restore each chakra to its optimum level of functioning. This means to heal the traumatized membranes so that the system has the opportunity to function optimally.

The first three chakras are really the crucible of the work with flower essences. It is here that the traumas and mishaps of our early lives lodge and do their work creating disease and unhappiness. The upper chakras are not considered until much later in the flower essence journey.

CHAKRA ONE: *Safety and Survival*

This is the lowest vibrating chakra. It is located below the base of the spine. It controls the distribution of energy to the entire physical structure. The health of the bones, the mineral content of the blood, the strength of the tissues, are all influenced by the health of the first chakra. It also influences the health of the lower spine, the colon, some functioning of the kidneys, the knees, feet, ankles and legs. The element associated with this chakra is earth. The color associated is a deep red or maroon. The color shifts from more red to more blue depending on the level of threat versus safety that the individual is experiencing.

When a child is born all chakras are functioning. The chakra system, however, is still connected to and part of the parents' energy systems. The developing child's chakras "go on line" or individualize as a separate system gradually as a part of the developmental process. What is happening is the individuality or soul-force of the child is gradually incarnating or coming into the chakra system. As this happens the chakra system is gradually infused with more and more of the individual's energy and less and less of the sustaining energy of the parents.

Chakra one begins its individualization process roughly around the time the child becomes upright and begins to walk. If the environment the child grows up in is safe — free from danger and hostility — if the child's physical and emotional needs are cared for properly, if there is no abuse, mistreatment or neglect of any kind, then chakra one is able to receive and hold the incoming soul force and development proceeds normally. Abuse, neglect, mistreatment, abandonment and negative imprinting all retard the development of this chakra and make it vulnerable to occupation by lower vibration. The low vibration of trauma prevents or delays the descent of soul force into the chakra. This makes the individual susceptible to fears and retards the development of the areas of the physical which are under the influence of this chakra, and makes these areas more vulnerable to disease.

Any danger, abuse, neglect, mistreatment or abandonment at any age can influence the health of this chakra. Most crucial, however, are the developmental years.

A healthy first chakra signals "all is well" throughout the system. This signal is necessary for rest, relaxation and rejuvenation and also to permit the individual to make the most out of fun and pleasure, energetic necessities to a healthy system.

Past trauma or conditioning can make it difficult for the chakra to produce this signal. Indeed, the experiences of the past where safety was breached make the system hyper-vigilant and more prone to physical, mental and emotional stresses. Those who are prone to constant worry, anxiety and fear can often point to safety issues in childhood.

This chakra is also keenly responsible for fight-flight responses. When there is a life-threatening situation or even a mild threat to the physical, such as touching something very hot, this chakra ignites the instinctive response toward self-preservation. It by-passes the rational decision-making process which is the domain of chakra three and commands the body to react.

Flower essences that treat this chakra will usually enhance a feeling of safety by raising the energy of the chakra. This will create a feeling of enhanced safety or a relief from a specific fear and give the person an opportunity to move the trauma out of the system more permanently.

This chakra has two essential signals. One tells the person that there is a threat to safety and the other tells the person that all is well—to relax. Nature provides these switches to protect and rejuvenate the system. Problems occur when signals from past threats interfere with the present reality. In a safe situation the person cannot relax or feels fear, or under threat, a person cannot respond.

Flower essences balance both of these situations. Black Cohosh, for instance, will help a person respond to the threat of being hurt by another, balancing the first chakra to provide stability and a healthy reflex. Blue Vervain will help a stressed person to relax by providing the signal of safety through the first chakra.

Flowers that influence this chakra tend to be from plants that have a blue color, a dark color, to grown low or downward, to be very large. Many trees support the first chakra.

CHAKRA TWO: *Relationship and Pleasure*

This chakra is located near the pelvic area. Through this chakra we develop an ability to have good healthy relationships with others. Through this center we also learn to accept or take in pleasure.

The second chakra influences the health of the reproductive system, the bladder, the pelvis, the fluids in the body. Its element is water. It is connected closely to the emotional body. Its color presents as a bluish-orange. More blue when at rest, peace or balance, more red to orange during threat or intense interaction.

Chakra two begins to individualize around the time of toilet training. This chakra is initially connected to the mother like an energetic umbilical cord. This energy cord stretches and weakens over the developmental period, finally (in a healthy relationship) breaking around the age of 17-20. There are several significant times in the development of this chakra: (generally) Age 2-3 when the child first expresses a difference of opinion from the parents; age 5-7 when the child goes to school; age 14-17 when the adolescent develops an identity away from the family and 18-20 when the child leaves home.

There are four independent actions of this chakra:

TO OPEN. This happens when the individual feels safe. Safety and trust are necessary for this action to occur. A more bluish color will flow through the chakra signaling it to open.

TO TAKE IN ENERGY. This happens when the chakra is open. Enjoyment, pleasure, fun, humor are all energetically similar. The second chakra is open and drawing in energy. This energy is stored and used by the system. The ability of the second chakra to draw in energy is a cornerstone of health. This ability is largely learned behavior. How a child is treated conditions this chakra to take in an amount of energy. One might call this function of the second chakra self-worth or worthiness. Tinges of yellow infuse the chakra during this function.

TO CLOSE. This happens when a person feels threat from others or another. This action is the initial reflex that stimulates the individuals protective system. More red-orange colors will occupy the chakra signaling the close. This red energy then surges upward in the chakra system making intense energy available for a healthy protective response.

TO CONNECT TO OTHERS. From this chakra we send out fibers or filaments that connect to others. Along these fibers we send and receive energy with others. The energetic contract of all relationships depends again on how healthy our parents were and on our indoctrination—what we learned about relationships from observation and experience.

A healthy second chakra possesses the instinctual capacity to close to threat and open to pleasure. It is able to take in energy in the form of pleasure and it forms healthy give and take relationships with others. Healthy parenting will insure a healthy functioning chakra. Poor parenting will retard or block this chakra's functioning. An individual with a retarded second chakra will have difficulty saying no, setting boundaries and maintaining healthy relationships.

There are several flowers here that influence this chakra. Motherwort, for instance, will help a person close the second chakra. This is helpful when past mistreatment prevents a person from being able to form healthy boundaries. Missouri Primrose helps a person to open this chakra and to take in energy. Missouri Primrose treats deep feelings of unworthiness which interfere with this process of taking in energy. Blackberry Lily will help a person process and release sexual trauma by stimulating the second chakra to increase *velocity*. Flowers treating the second chakra tend to be orange or yellow. Cuplike yellow flowers and the lily family are also resonant with this chakra and relationship issues.

CHAKRA THREE: *Identity, Integration, Will Forces, Manifestation*

The third chakra sits in the area of the solar plexus. Its element is fire. Its color is flame-like ranging from blue to yellow-white. It distributes energy throughout the rhythmic systems, which include the circulatory system and the lungs. It is connected to the mental body and left-brain thinking. This chakra begins to individualize as soon as the child has learned to close the second chakra. This begins when the child learns to say "no."

This chakra has two primary functions:

INTEGRATION AND IDENTITY. Chakra three collects information from other chakras into understandable wholes. Our sense of what is real comes through the integration work of this chakra. It assembles various parts of the self from all of the information from the past and present contained in the chakra system, and creates a sense of self or identity.

WILL FORCES AND MANIFESTATION. While chakra two draws in energy, chakra three projects energy outward into the world. When we think, plan and perform actions, we are using this chakra. The initial reflex is usually mental. We think about what we will do. As we do this, energy streams from this chakra and begins to create an energetic glove, which our actions then fit into. The next reflex is the action itself. We are always creating our lives energetically and then entering the field we have projected. This is why creative visualization works to the extent it does.

What we call circumstance, that is, those things that *happen* to us, are in fact results of *emanations* from this energy center. Many of these are conscious, but some of them proceed from our subconscious. This means chakra three projects out our plans, hopes and dreams as well as our fears. These projections bring people, things, events and circumstance to us. This function has been traditionally relegated to chance, but in fact happens through the activity of our consciousness acting through this chakra.

The energy used by chakra three is the energy that is taken in by chakra two. These two chakras working together comprise the mechanism we call self-esteem. The first part of this is worthiness, self-acceptance, self-love. This is the quality that allows chakra two to draw in energy. This energy is taken up to chakra three where it is projected out in the form of confidence, the second part of self-esteem.

The more energy that is taken in, the more that is available for use; the less taken in, the less available. This means that those who do not allow themselves to play or to enjoy, eventually find themselves without energy. Another way of saying this is "all work and no play can lead to depression and burnout."

Problems in manifestation or creating the life one wants come about largely because both conscious and unconscious energy are circulating through chakras two and three. In other words a person not only puts out into the world what he or she wants consciously, but also the ill experiences or imprints of the past that are, perhaps, buried are being projected out, bringing the *familiar* into one's life.

This is energetically how history repeats itself in our lives or how, for instance, people find themselves married to partners reminding them of their parents.

Most daisies will influence this chakra. For instance, Elecampagne, a yellow daisy, will help a person take in new information about the self more quickly, thereby accelerating the growth, development or recovery process.

THE RED AND BLUE CHANNELS
Links Between the Chakras

Connecting the chakras are two main channels or highways. The red channel conducts red energy upward and the blue conducts blue energy downward. Red energy is used in situations of threat, while the blue energy circulates during times of safety. At any moment both energies are circulating through the system. In most situations, one energy predominates. All chakras become more red or more blue depending on which energy is circulating through the system.

When an individual senses threat, the first chakra telegraphs a signal to the second chakra which closes and begins to send red energy upward. All chakras become more red in color. This energy is used essentially to protect the individual from harm. This red energy can be seen easily when one is angry. The chest, neck and face turn red. The entire body is prepared to express a forceful energy to end the threat. The more intense the threat, the more intense the response. Blocking the expressions of anger that the red channel carries causes many health problems. Many inflammations are the result of repressed red energy that still circulate through the system.

This red channel is activated when a person is working under stress. The threat of being late or not completing a task or fear of failure, and so on, cause a person to engage this system in normal daily routines of work or child care or task management. This channel is intended by nature to be used occasionally, not all the time. Activating the red channel frequently can cause health problems.

When the first chakra senses "all is well," it tells the system to relax, enjoy, wind down for restoration. When this happens, all the chakras become a little more blue. In this state, pulse, blood pressure and respiration all drop and the system is prepared to rest or to sleep. Problems occur when fears do not permit the first chakra to send the "all is well" signal to switch on. Indeed, in the world today with the many ever-present threats, it is more and more a challenge to access this state of safety and relaxation.

Blue Vervain, Lemon Balm and Blue Lobelia stimulate the blue channel; Motherwort, Mountain Pride or Red Monkeyflower stimulate the red channel.

How flower essences work energetically is to create a *temporary* change or shift in the chakra system. This change will allow the individual *more choice*. As the individual makes healthier choices, the chakra system holds its temporary configuration and the flower essence is no longer needed. This process may take a short or a long time depending on many variables in a person's history and support system, but it is essentially unique to this field — flower essences assist with healthy choice and healthy choice changes the individual.

A Note on Preparation and Dosage

The standard format for this section is the number of drops of stock essence per 100 drops of neutral solution. Neutral solution here means a brandy-water solution bottle that is prepared to receive a certain number of drops of the stock essence for the treatment bottle or dosage bottle as it is called by many practitioners. Since practitioners use different size bottles for treatment, I felt it best to be more precise in explaining the best level to prepare each essence.

There are roughly 340 drops in a half-ounce bottle and almost 700 in a full-ounce bottle. Adding 3 drops to a half-ounce bottle is about 1 drop per 100 and adding 7 drops to a one-ounce bottle is about 1 drop per 100. The dosage given under the preparation and dosage heading for each flower is, in my research, the one that yields the best results.

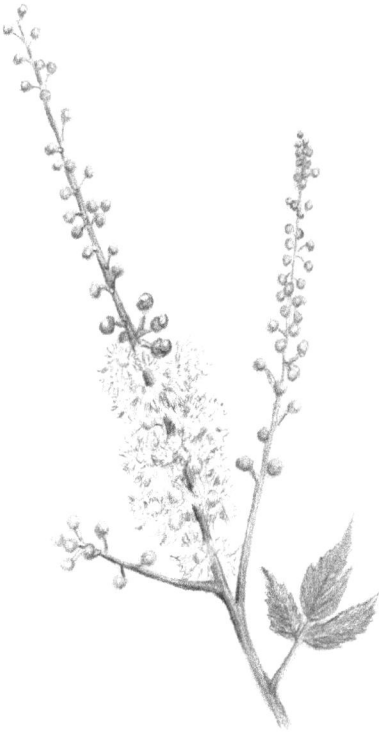

BLACK COHOSH

Cimicifuga racemosa

No harm comes to me.

The Black Cohosh plant itself is a paradox. It grows in the deep eastern woods of the United States. The contrast between the black root and the white flowers along with its ability to grow tall spikes in the shade make this an unusual plant, indeed. Traditionally, Black Cohosh, as an herb, treats the uterus and the spine. It relaxes the central nervous system, eases pelvic symptoms, and helps with head and neck tensions, including migraines. The homeopathic treatment is similar but adds a dark, brooding, depressive personality type as an indication for treatment.

Indications: Has lower back problems; fears being hurt; fears loud voices; fears strong personalities; fears violence; has prostate problems; has stiff neck; is caught in abusive relationships; feels victimized; attracts dark personalities; acts the role of peacekeeper; feels heavy depression; dreams of being trapped; dreams of being pursued by vague dark forces.

Black Cohosh, in its most basic application is a remedy that treats a primal fear—the fear of violence or of being hurt by others. Although this usually means strong, aggressive, ruthless people, the fear can be generalized to include many other types. Although violence inspires a healthy and natural level of fear, the fear in question is an irrational, skewed reflex—not to violence itself but to stimuli that imply violence to the person such as strength, loudness, crassness, or any specific personality type or situation.

Violence in one's history skews the personality in many ways. The most direct and obvious way is when there has been an angry, violent, aggressive personality in one's history, one then fears and avoids this type of person into adulthood. Less direct, is the personality that avoids the experience of anger altogether, cutting off even the inner impulses of anger, outrage or aggression, even when they are appropriate and called for. In both cases, Black Cohosh, in its ability to treat the underlying fears, helps to balance the personality to be able to include a healthier range of responses to strong personalities.

Another, and not so obvious, way that the personality adapts in response to violence in its history, is to become attracted to violent or dark personalities. It is as if the personality of the victim has split and cannot function properly in response to potential harm. One part sees possible danger while another cannot resist being enchanted by or drawn to it. Some people have several close relationships with dark, violent perpetrators before coming to grips with the reality that one is living a diminished life in a kind of captivity. Sometimes the perpetrator has a charming side which further complicates the deception and darkens the shadow the victim lives within. Here, Black Cohosh provides clarity, lifting the spell, and showing people and situations for what they are and not what they pretend to be.

Black Cohosh is a tonic for timidity and fear of confrontations. There is a strengthening that happens with this essence that allows a person to remain engaged in dialogue, conflict, or negotiation without a reflex to avoid or disengage. Here it is best that the client take the essence with a particular person or confrontation in mind. In this way the shifting becomes more obvious and practical.

Black Cohosh is also recommended when a person *attracts* dark or violent personalities unconsciously. Here the person responds to malevolence in a healthy way once there is a recognition. The problem, however, is that these dark personality types keep showing up and making their presence known. With Black Cohosh there is a reckoning with the unconscious aspects that are attracting these unwanted types and an easing of the problem.

Black Cohosh flower essence can be beneficial for lower back, neck, or pelvic issues when the subject has some of the fears or issues mentioned here. The Black Cohosh type will have: 1. a harmful or violent caregiver in his or her past; 2. some above-mentioned personality issues; 3. some physical issues in the lower back, neck, pelvic area, or head.

Energetically, Black Cohosh stimulates the first chakra directly adding velocity to sluggish areas. These darker areas lower the vibration of the chakra making the individual more vulnerable to fears. This type of restriction in the first chakra will prevent a person from making connections with the cords or emanating fibers of the second chakra. As the first chakra becomes less impeded there is less strain on the sphincter muscle allowing the spine and central nervous system to work more fluidly and efficiently. This is how the essence can influence problems in the spine, especially with this personality type.

Use Black Cohosh with children who are afraid of loud or strong personalities. This might be men with deep voices or women with high shrill voices. Use it also for children who fear certain hats or uniforms. A single application of Black Cohosh can make a noticeable difference.

Use Black Cohosh with animals who are at the bottom of the pecking order. This applies to horses, dogs, cats, and birds. If possible, make the essence available to the victim pet only, and for a period of one week to ten days. Use in the same way for dogs who react to loud or deep voices.

Preparation and dosage: Add one drop of stock solution per 100 drops of neutral solution. Use the stock solution when treating physical symptoms. Add one drop of stock solution to 700 drops of neutral solution when doing past life work.

See also: Motherwort, Black Currant, Hemp Agrimony, Gravel Root.

BLACK CURRANT

Ribes nigrum

I am here, I am real, I exist.

Currants are berries that grow in hedges or bushes. They have both nutritional and medicinal value, being high in vitamins B and C, and astringent in herbal use.

Indications: Fears abandonment; fears death; feels invisible; feels slighted or ignored easily; fears not existing; fears being in crowds; fears ending relationships; fears competition; has unexplained fears and anxiety; resists change; feels dread; expects failure; possesses a general existential gloom; is agnostic; fears risk; fears change in general; is cynical; secretly denies metaphysical realities; tends towards extreme materialism; is over-rational.

The human soul thrives in an atmosphere of loving, caring attention. The healthy ego or sense of self is formed when these energies abound; likewise, in their absence, the self struggles and flounders. A healthy ego is necessary for taking risks and making change. When, because of neglect or abandonment, the ego is poorly formed, it becomes vulnerable to many fears, especially those that threaten the experience of the self.

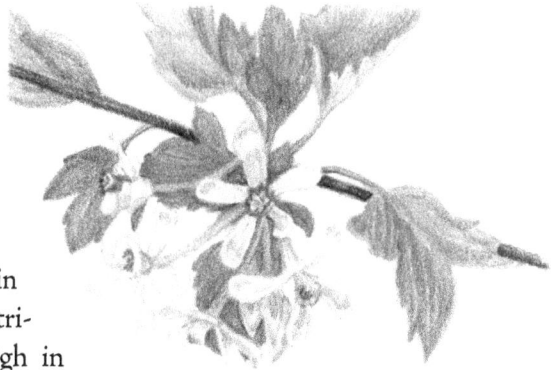

Black Currant flower essence addresses a deep fear in the soul, the fear of non-existence, or not being. This fear is largely unconscious and gains its power from its hidden nature. It surfaces when one experiences events that threaten the self or when those people, places, and things that define the self change or go away. Whenever we make a major change the self, in a sense, diminishes.

Adults who are doing work to heal aspects of the personality confront this fear when they realize, as the self changes, that they are not the parts of the personality that they have identified within the past as the "self." This fear arises when the finite mind realizes that it cannot grasp who the "self" is. This is sometimes the case when one does deep transformational work and has a breakthrough, or when one enters an unfamiliar but expanded state. The former sense of "self" cannot contain the new experience and has not developed a new reference point. This experience can trigger this otherwise unconscious fear.

Often when there is a deep and authentic experience of a spiritual nature, especially one that challenges previous beliefs, an individual reacts by escaping into a kind of subconscious denial. Some symptoms which characterize this state are: an increase in addictive behavior, inability to focus on mundane matters which previously held the individual's interest, difficulty sleeping, a decrease in tolerance thresholds, an increase in cynicism. It is as if part of the personality is trying to grasp the intensity of the experience, while another part is trying to forget that it happened. Black Currant gives both the courage and illumination needed to look at and integrate this new experience and the new meaning of "self" that the experience carries.

Today there are deep and profound questions about life and death that are no longer culturally or simplistically explained, but are lurking in the subconscious and can bring about unrest and anxiety, especially at transition times in one's life, if they are not confronted. Black Currant gives the soul the courage to go beyond this internal fear and conflict in order to continue its journey into truth, light, and the meaning of eternity.

Fears of abandonment are eased with this essence. Those who have trouble ending relationships or moving on to new phases in their lives, hanging on to the old, will find a new courage in ending the old and accepting the new.

Black Currant helps those who are disoriented or express timidity after an experience of growth or expansion. Use it with children who become obsessively anxious over death — especially after the death of a pet or a loved one, or who become fearful after a major family change. Black Currant helps with midlife crises or with major change in behavior, attitude, or habits in adults. It is a useful essence for animals of owners who have a preoccupation with fears of death. These individuals often use their pets for observation and reflection about life and death. Black Currant, in this case, helps animals remain free from the stress and fears that surround such individuals.

Use this essence to comfort the fears of those who are dying and do not believe in the survival of the soul or personality after death. It can ease the overwhelming dread and the incapacitating fear that accompanies this type of transition.

Energetically, this essence works with the inner or deeper energies of the first three chakras (the domain of the inner child) giving added light and higher vibration. When chakra three develops — the identity chakra — it relies on the strength of the lower two for its healthy formation. Abandonment and neglect create a weakened structure for the identity to develop, resulting in an ego structure that cannot withstand the normal stresses of risk and change. The ego receives added energy with this essence and therefore strength and freedom from fears.

Preparation and Dosage: Add one drop of stock essence per 300 drops of neutral solution for general treatment; use one drop per 100 when treating conscious fears, anxieties, and resistance, especially when the individual has gone through intense personal changes.

See Also: Elecampagne, Indian Tobacco.

BLACKBERRY LILY

Belamcanda chinensis

My relationships are filled with clarity and joy.

Blackberry Lily is also called Candy Lily or Chinese Lily. It blooms in late summer and produces seeds that look like black-berries. The spotted orange flowers are small and twist into tightly packed clusters. This herb is used in Chinese medicine for asthma, wheezing, sore throats and bronchitis. Externally it has been used in western herbalism for sprains, boils, contusions and as a remedy for breast cancer.

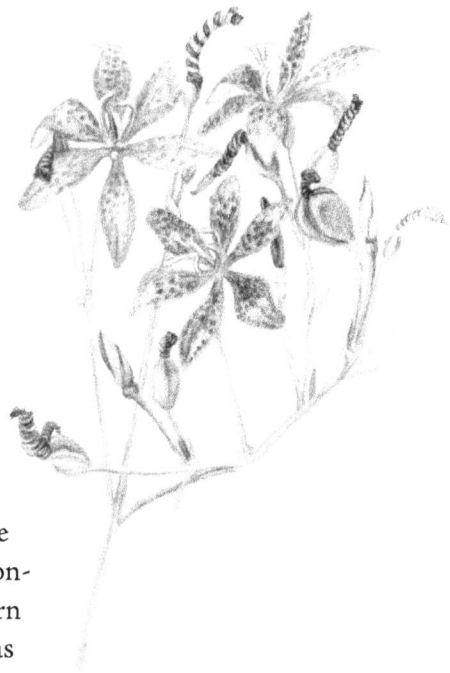

Indications: Feels victimized; relives old patterns in new relationships; fears relationship; feels betrayal by partners and friends; is unable to attract or maintain healthy relationships; fears closeness; has strong gender related attitudes; attracts drama; has symptoms of: infertility, endometriosis, uterine tumors, bladder infections, sexual imbalances, genital inflammations, genital rashes or lower back problems.

This essence helps heal and balance many aspects of friendship, love and sexuality, especially when something repressed in the psyche is skewing one's experience of others. Our subconscious in this case fuels the imagination to create dynamics and circumstances which appear to be real on the surface, but are in actuality our own creation. The psyche is in reality dancing to music of the past, which the conscious mind cannot hear but can only observe the results.

One example of this might be in a relationship where one partner has had previous sexual trauma, which is interfering with a healthy sexual relationship between partners. Often it will appear as if it is a dynamic between the two — that both are responsible for the difficulty. While in one sense this is true, the most obscure and potent dynamic is often the repressed information of the partner who has experienced the trauma. It is useful in this case for both partners to take the essence, although some benefit will be achieved if either one takes it.

Although treatment for repressed trauma is a common use for this essence, its general action is much more universal in treating any subconscious imprint interfering with objectivity about relationships of all types. Blackberry Lily helps bring the information needed forward to the conscious mind and for this reason complements any counseling process, especially couples therapy.

Those needing the essence may feel trapped, fated or cursed to have bad relationships or no relationships at all or they complain about seeing the same cycle occur over and over with different partners or close friends. Or there may be negative gender related attitudes.

Energetically, the second chakra gains velocity when one takes this essence. This acceleration initially throws lower frequencies lodged in the chakra out and into the circulating energy system. When this happens, the conscious mind now has access to information that was previously unavailable. The dark spots in this lily are a significant part of the language of the flower since trauma generally appears as darker areas in the chakra. This coloring of the flower creates a sympathy with traumatized areas of the chakra. When using this essence watch for changes or temporary aggravations in somatized pelvic symptoms or lower back difficulties.

Blackberry Lily is useful for past life work when some event from another lifetime is interfering with relationships in the present incarnation. Preschool children who express strong instinctive dislikes for certain other children can benefit from this essence. Animals who exhibit sudden and latent antisocial behavior often have accessed a repressed imprint in someone in the household and could benefit from Blackberry Lily. Although it is ideal for both the household member and animal to take the essence, it is most often the case that the stewards of animals are entirely unaware that the imprint causing the animal behavior is coming from inside them.

Preparation and Dosage: Two drops of stock essence per 100 drops of neutral solution; four drops if the person has therapeutic support and is working on past sexual trauma. Use the stock bottle to treat somatized pelvic symptoms.

See Also: Wood Betony, Star Jasmine, Pink Amaranthus, Gravel Root, Hemp Agrimony, Butterflyweed, Milk Thistle.

BLESSED THISTLE

Carduus benedictus

God is Love.

One of the most beautiful of the thistles, the flowers are red and golden appearing in the summer. Also named "Holy Thistle" for the many benefits derived from the plant. Although cultivated for centuries in this country, it is native to southern Europe where it is found in waste, stony and uncultivated areas. The entire plant is used medicinally. It benefits the digestive system, purifies the blood, stimulates circulation, and is useful for all liver problems. It is a remedy for fevers and as a tonic, it strengthens the heart, brain and stomach.

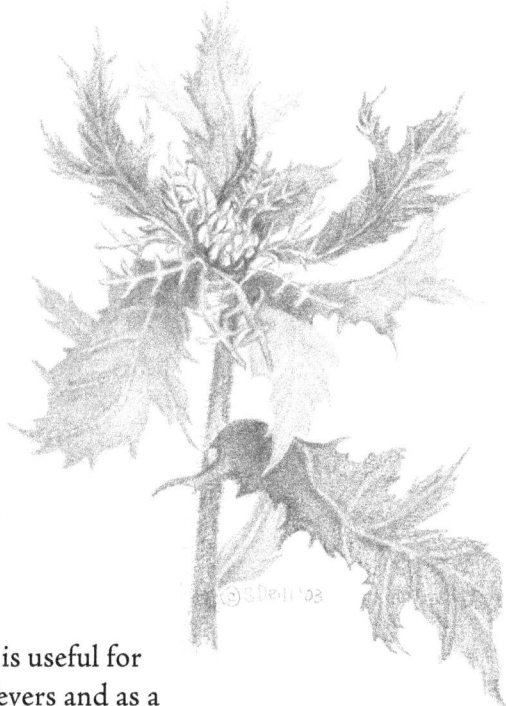

Indications: Fears fate, destiny or the hand of God; feels that God and nature are essentially cruel; fears power; is unable to flow with life; attracts overbearing personality types; has agnostic or atheistic beliefs; was abused by father figure; needs to control; is over-insured; has problems with prostate; headaches; agoraphobia; fears heights; fears dying; is angry or confused in the face of disappointment or tragedy; fears law enforcement or establishment.

Blessed Thistle flower essence helps to ease a fear of life or of the Forces that guide all things. It is not as though a person fears God as such, but can have a deep abiding fear of the "Hand of God" or a trepidation of the cruelty or impersonal nature of fate. There are many things that can cause such a fear in a person: guilt, experiences of bad luck or tragedy, philosophies absorbed from parents, background or indoctrination into some religions. Blessed Thistle eases these fears, helping a person to be more able to flow with life, accepting the possibility of earthly happiness.

The concept of a loving God is a comparatively recent development in many religions. There is still a widespread belief in a God of retribution and punishment. This belief runs deep in the collective soul of humankind, giving many the convenient interpretation of Divine Intervention as an explanation of the many terrible events that occur in the world today. For some then, God must be punishing us for something; for others God must not exist at all; for still others there is only an intellectual or surface belief that God is Good, Loving and Present.

At each failure, disappointment and tragedy in life, the human soul reaches to grasp the meaning of such pain amidst the belief in the presence of a Loving Creator. This journey is part of the evolution of the human soul, as we must resolve *experientially* the paradox of a loving God with the presence of tragedy and evil in the world. Blessed Thistle flower essence helps the individual soul to resume the journey of the soul to God by easing many of the fears, doubts and misgivings we have been taught or have developed regarding God's relationship to the human race and to the individual.

Within this scope, Blessed Thistle can have many effects on the psyche. For clergy, it can help with the little doubts that creep into the corner of the soul. For atheists, it can help with blocks to mental clarity which are caused by fear and helplessness and which twist the powers of observation and logic or intensify the denial of facts, which may refute their case. It can help the very materialistic open to possibilities of other levels of satisfaction. For many, there is a reawakening of possibilities for relationship with God and an acceptance of the experience of God's Love in their hearts and in their lives.

Another effect of Blessed Thistle flower essence is a renewal of the ability to flow with life — to see more clearly how God is working with us. It is far less difficult to flow with life when we are certain that the powers that control our lives are wise and loving in nature. Blessed Thistle prepares the individual for a deeper, more interactive and more profound relationship with the Divine.

Blessed Thistle is helpful at various stages in the spiritual development process. There can be fears and doubts that arise on the heels of an authentic and profound experience of the Divine. There can be a waning of enthusiasm or a period of retreat from an active pursuit of spiritual goals. The essence here acts very quickly in helping the pilgrim resume the journey with conviction and eagerness.

Energetically, there is a harmonization of the first two chakras to receive energies from the crown. In other words, the chakras will develop a similar vibration and thereby "talk" better to each other. This assists the journey of resolution between the divine and animal natures. One learns the practical and personal meaning of the Divine.

Blessed Thistle is another essence that is useful for hospice workers. It can help the individual who is passing to feel a closer connection to God. It can help family members feel more the mystery and love associated with this process than the fear and the sadness.

Children enjoy Blessed Thistle during times when their developing minds come to grips with some of the deeper questions about the existence and nature of God. It is best here if the parent or caregiver takes the essence along with the child for a day or two while the questions and the answers are alive in the soul.

Animals feel very quickly the effects of Blessed Thistle. It is useful for general household stress that may be transferred to the animal. It is especially useful for animals to take when there is a death in the family. Dying animals are given added comfort with this essence.

Preparation and Dosage: Add one drop of stock essence per 100 drops of neutral solution for adults, children and animals. Use one drop per 1000 in a spray in homes where someone is dying or has passed recently. Apply the spray every three hours.

See Also: Golden Amaranthus, Indian Tobacco.

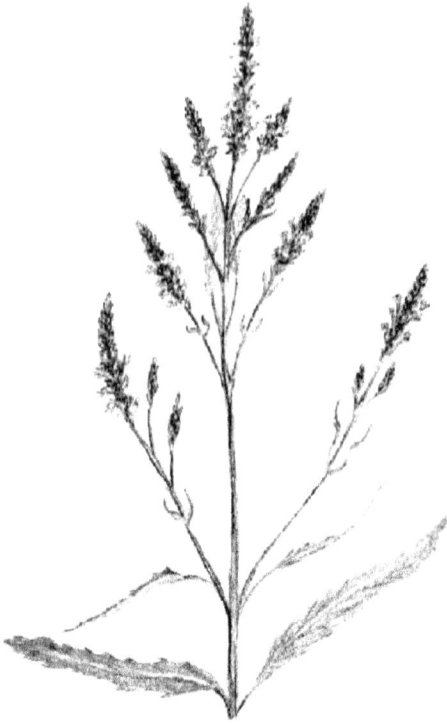

BLUE VERVAIN

Verbena hastate

I am safe in the power of love.

Also known as Wild Hyssop, Blue Vervain is indigenous to the United States. According to Matthew Wood, a prominent North American herbalist, it is still used by Native American practitioners as a nervine and an antispasmodic. The signature of the plant is its intense blue flowers and square stems, indicating nerves. Flowers, leaves and stems are used medicinally. It may treat muscle spasms in the neck and shoulders; it is used also as a relaxant and to reduce fevers.

Indications: Has difficulty sleeping; thinks obsessively; has headaches, eye problems, dizziness, neck tension, weak ankles, weak knees, or digestive problems; is a workaholic; has sluggish kidneys or stones, heartburn, nightmares, unable to relax; neglects taking care of self; has difficulty socializing; acts aloof or unfriendly.

Blue Vervain flower essence is an ideal remedy for mental stress. It eases the brutal effect the busy mind can have over the body when focused mental forces produce intense directed energy. At first the intensity and the focus of the mind overwhelms the needs of the body. Over time the energy becomes destructive to the physical.

Now and then, most of us are faced with challenges that demand such intense focus and energy that we temporarily ignore or neglect some very basic physical needs. We may, for a period of time, forget about food, sleep and other basic needs because of a more overwhelming need to achieve some important goal. Emergencies, deadlines, competitions and disasters are examples of situations that are likely to inspire this type of condition of high alert and maximum output. Many agree that the very best in human potential occurs during these times.

Problems, however, can arise both in the body and mind when this type of energy becomes a lifestyle or a hallmark of the personality. In this case the individual seeks situations that demand a high intensity of dedication and involvement. Over time, the body begins to react to this type of subjugation, becoming stressed and depleted, losing resistance to disease. Stress, anxiety and types of addictions that calm the nerves become common. Blue Vervain treats personalities that are driven and regularly use mental or physical forces, and push, dominate, even punish their bodies. In some cases the subjugation is conscious and deliberate, in others it is unconscious and a by-product of the intense involvement with the situation or work at hand.

Need for Blue Vervain in the present day is very high. One part of the problem is social. Images and ideas of success will induce many to sacrifice or invest a period of their lives to achieve whatever feels like success. Core social-economic values will reward the driven personality in most areas of industry, politics, military or religion. It is more common for a "go-getter" to be sought out or rewarded than a balanced, even personality. Society today respects, rewards, seeks, cultivates and supports the driven personality without concern or awareness that this type of personality is on a direct course with some significant health problems.

Another part of the problem is psychological. The line between dedication to work and workaholism is thin. The same neglect/abuse to the physical can be present in both. As society at large becomes more sensitive to addictive behavior and more sophisticated in its treatments, this aspect is likely to decrease.

Energetically, Blue Vervain's color is key to its effect on the system. It strengthens the "downward" or blue channel interchange between the chakras. This channel connects with the coolness of the first or earth chakra. This chakra, in turn, feeds the physical body by directly signaling vibrations of safety and is responsible for our ability to sense physical needs. In an alert or "overdrive" condition, the red or "upward" channel works intensely, dwarfing the ability of the blue channel to cool or ease the nervous systems and the inner organs. The results of this are some common symptoms of this kind of stress: tightness in the upper back and shoulders, eye strain, headaches, inflammations from the neck up (e.g., sore eyes, rashes on the face and scalp, or earaches); weakness in the lower body, sluggish kidneys or stones, weakness or pain in the knees or ankles. Blue Vervain treats all of these symptoms especially in this type of personality.

Taken over time, Blue Vervain flower essence will balance the driven personality who can then learn other ways of approaching life, completing tasks — other paradigms for success. It is best taken when the individual is beginning to realize that the program s/he is running may not be in his/her best interests.

This usually means realizing that the problems being experienced with physical and mental health have something to do with the personality.

Those who are workaholics will find this essence helpful for recovering from their addictive behavior. In this case, energy to the emotional chakra is often being blocked, the upward energy conveniently avoiding contact with the second chakra. Blue Vervain flower essence's cooling downward energy gently resets the pathways, making it easier to access emotions that are being shut out of the system. Working with a good therapist while taking the essence will accelerate the recovery process.

Animals such as horses, who are intensely trained for show or racing or dogs who guide or guard, will relax more deeply during "down time" with this essence, and will be better able to deal with the high stress of their jobs.

Firstborn children, high-achieving children or children of high-achieving parents will learn to deal better with daily stresses with this essence.

Preparation and Dosage: Add one drop of stock essence per 100 drops of neutral solution. Add 10 drops of stock essence per 100 drops neutral solution to treat physical symptoms arising from stress. For animals, add one drop of stock per 200 drops of neutral solution.

See Also: Golden Amaranthus, Lemon Balm.

BORAGE

Borago officinalis

I feel courage, strength, and joy.

The name Borage is derived from the Celtic word "*barrach,*" meaning "man of courage." Many historical references are made regarding Borage being effective in raising the spirits, comforting the heart and promoting a general feeling of happiness. The leaves and flowers are used medicinally. In addition to its ability to reduce fevers and provide anti-inflammatory action in pulmonary conditions, it has a definite tonic effect on the adrenals, known in Chinese medicine as the "organ of courage."

Indications: Is shy, reluctant, withdrawn; feels dread; is downcast, bored or desperate; fears failure; fears confrontation or conflict; fears hurting others; feels sad, depressed, hopeless or tired of one's life; has stomach problems; has adrenal

imbalances; feels suicidal; feels
that life is empty or meaningless;
feels stuck or cursed; feels afraid
to make changes.

This is a powerful and versa-
tile essence with many uses. The
entire plant radiates a celebration
of life and for this reason has
been called the "herb of glad-
ness." Its joyfulness attracts
the soul force more deeply
into the physical. This is
especially useful during
times of challenge when the
light of incarnation has been
displaced by sadness, turmoil or
worry. During these times we are
likely to feel our own heaviness.
Life force cannot circulate properly
and we find ourselves feeling empty,
limp and joyless.

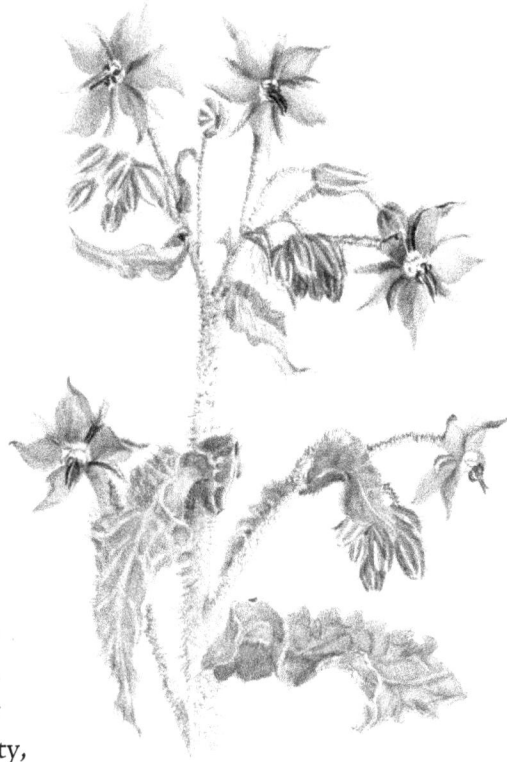

This condition happens frequently
today and for many reasons. Borage excels when one feels burdened by the
recurring daily events of life that tax the soul. Overwork, feeling trapped, failure, repetition, frustration are some of the ways we fall victim to being downcast in this way.

At times during some depressions, the longing to be free from this condition moves the soul to the unconscious for solutions. Among the solutions
entertained by the unconscious is to leave incarnation. Although there may be
no conscious wish at all to leave, the frustrations of the conscious mind yield to
despair and the unconscious impulses take over. Borage gives a feeling of presence, groundedness, embodiment, even stoutheartedness to assist the conscious
mind in choosing to stay in incarnation and to have hope.

Energetically, Borage stimulates both a downward and upward movement
in the chakra system. The downward movement activates a movement of soul-
force into the lower chakras. This movement strengthens a feeling of solidity,
enhancing incarnation. At the same time, the flower coaxes movement upward
and into the solar plexus. Individuality and commitment are renewed. A person
is likely to see a gradual development of empowerment and goal-directed

behavior. These, in turn, become part of the antidote for the state of defeat, helplessness and powerlessness.

Dogs who are depressed or begin showing patterns of sleeping more or changes in eating habits in response to being left unattended for long periods can benefit from Borage, as would sensitive animals who lose vigor during times of suppressed turmoil in the human family, such as dogs or cats who become lethargic when their owners are in a period of not speaking to each other out of anger.

Grammar school-aged children who do not like school would enjoy Borage. This can mean either children who are afraid of school, or those who become bored and apathetic because of the monotony and repetition. In addition, adults who are challenged by their jobs, financial stress or relationships, and feel occasionally disheartened would like this essence.

Use Borage also in combinations that promote emotional release. It significantly relieves the intensity of the feeling of loss of energy or hope, which sometimes accompanies deep processing.

Preparation and Dosage: Add one drop of stock essence per 100 drops of neutral solution. Take a few drops of this 2-3 times a day.

See Also: Star Jasmine, Motherwort, Lemon Balm, Horseradish.

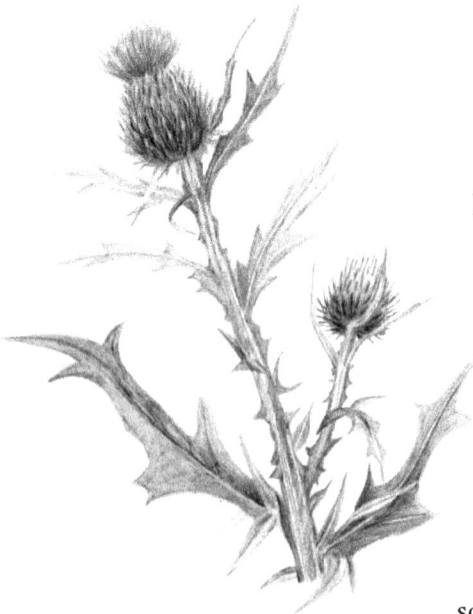

BULL THISTLE

Cirsium vulgaris

I am free.

Bull Thistle is an annual herb with sharp, star-shaped leaves and reddish flowers that bloom in the summer. The airborne seeds of Bull Thistle tend to make it invasive to some gardeners and farmers. It has been used herbally to treat inflammations.

Indications: Is claustrophobic, rebellious, insubordinate; has problems with authority; fears being controlled by others; has some types of paranoia; has an obsessive involvement with causes; is anti-social; is ultra-individualistic; fears socialism; dreams of being chased, caught, restrained or buried; is resistant to structure.

Although a certain amount of structure is vital for all phases of growth and development, many institutions—parenting, schools, religions, the workplace—have, especially in the past, imposed stringent controls that retard growth and have a negative effect on the psyche. It can be, for instance, that an individual, because of early experiences with a controlling parent, later in life rebels against all structures and has unconsciously developed attitudes and philosophies that are essentially anti-structure. There can also be irrational fears of being controlled that interfere with healthy membership in structured groups or organizations.

Bull Thistle assists the individual in releasing negative past experiences with structure or authority. The cleansing of these imprints allows the individual more freedom and choices as a member of groups of all kinds. Although a healthy skepticism remains, the individual is more able to see situations clearly and to trust healthy structures and leaders.

This essence also helps to ease fears of being controlled or confined even to the obsessive level. Use this essence for those who are claustrophobic, who fear being in crowds or who have recurring nightmares of being restrained, smothered, drowned or buried. Bull Thistle helps in various stages of recovery from rape, torture or imprisonment, especially when the individual is either wishing to change present behaviors and feelings, or is in touch with fearful memories for the first time. This essence can help with relationship or sexual therapy when one or both partners has been restrained and abused in the past. It is helpful for adults who were tied by parents with leashes or ropes as children.

Bull Thistle can soften those who exercise authority harshly, especially when such practices are related to fears of losing control. For example, supervisors who are new or insecure about their abilities to lead others might benefit from this essence.

Energetically, the action of Bull Thistle is mostly in chakra three, which has absorbed some primal fears which have not been held in check by the first chakra. These fears generally cannot be experienced directly because of their overpowering intensity. Instead they "leak" into other parts of the system and can skew emotions, thinking and behavior, or cause nightmares. A healthy birth and childhood will generally protect the personality from these fears. Bull Thistle eases these fears by first clearing the mental body (attached to chakra three) and then by strengthening the first chakra to keep these imprints out of the system.

This essence is helpful for children who excessively challenge or rebel against rules, authority and schedules. It is a general tonic for adolescent and teenage rebelliousness. Use Bull Thistle to relieve the stress of confinement for all animals, especially dogs bred close to ancestral strains of wolves. It is also helpful for caged birds, pet rodents and turtles.

Preparation and Dosage: Add one drop of stock essence per 100 drops of neutral solution. Apply three drops of this 3-5 times per day; more often when fears are present.

See Also: Butterfly Weed.

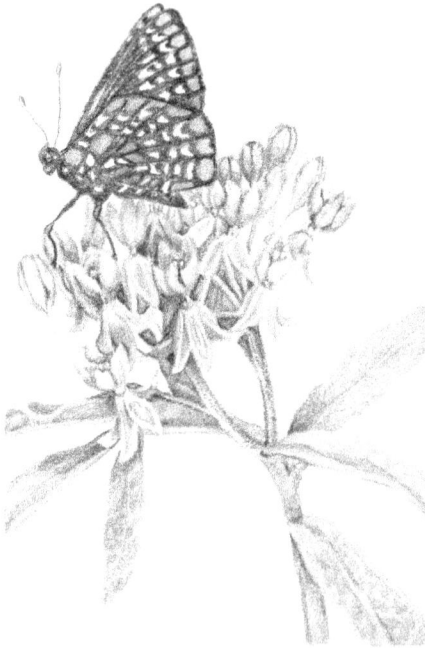

BUTTERFLY WEED

Asclepias tuberosa

I am free to love.

This small- to medium-sized plant is a bright orange color, attracting butterflies in the summertime. A relative to the Milkweed, it develops seedpods which open to spread flying seeds with the wind in the autumn. Butterflyweed appears later in the spring than most plants, its dramatic appearance often a surprise. Also called Pleurisy Root, this plant has been used for lung inflammations, asthma, bronchitis, bruises, swellings and rheumatism.

Indications: Fears commitment; avoids relationships; is love addicted; has boundary problems; has problems with sexual excess, impotency, or frigidity; has anger attacks or panic attacks; fears being in relationships; has urinary problems; bickers; gossips; is unfaithful; has obsessive sexual fantasies; tends to smother or be aloof in relationships.

This flower essence works with two dynamics in the personality: love and freedom. You might say that in order to love, one must resolve the apparent paradox between these two ideals. On one hand, the feeling of love is very liberating in itself; on the other hand, love involves commitment and giving of one's self, which can be seen and experienced as a loss of freedom. Love also means allowing the other person to be free. Every individual who loves others or another must at some point come to terms with this paradox and create a balance between these two great forces of human development.

The term, "love addiction," today refers to those who are so drawn to the "high" of the initial stages of being in love, that they end one relationship after another, feeling disappointment and frustration when the initial infatuation begins to ebb. Often the person agonizes about the feeling being gone as if some mysterious force or cruel hand of fate actually removes it. What is happening here, in most cases, is that there is a fear of entering deeper levels of relationship. This causes the person to subconsciously withdraw from the love feelings. The fear here, in most cases, is either of being hurt or of being trapped. Butterflyweed flower essence eases these fears, allowing for more maturity and deeper relationship. Like other addictions, love addiction requires other interventions such as counseling and support groups.

Adults who, as children, had the experience of parents who were boundary-invasive or smothering can also have issues within this polarity of love and freedom. There can be a dynamic of almost simultaneous attraction and repulsion when one, with a history of a smothering parent, chooses a similar personality type for a partner. On one hand, the person feels safe because of the strong personality of the partner; on the other hand, there can be a need for distance or to rebel or to hurt the other person. Butterflyweed here helps the adult to be more conscious of the difference between love and dependence.

This essence evens and balances the action of the second chakra. This regular rhythm can assist those who use the intensified action of the second chakra for an escape. The evenness of the movement interferes with the tendency to speed up the rhythm of the chakra to create addictive "highs." The closing action of the second chakra is enhanced by this stabilizing action. Intense velocities connected to emotional or sexual highs interfere with the ability of the individual to close this chakra to set boundaries with others. This means that the basis for creating relationship or energetic connection with others can change dramatically. For this reason, this essence works well with many types of relationship therapy, and should be considered for all adolescents and teens who are beginning to date.

In improving the balance of boundaries between one's self and others, this essence can help with general ease in relationships, removing the potential for regular confrontation or conflict. It can also help with anger attacks or panic attacks when the basis for these is boundary issues.

This is an excellent essence to take during family or couples therapy. It is good for children who are generally dependent and needy. It is helpful for early stages of psychotherapy, helping clients to remain conscious of any parental issues that are being transferred onto the therapist. It can help with resistance to toilet training, especially when a new baby is born into the family just before or during the training period.

When problems arise between sexual partners, this essence can very often be helpful. This is especially true when issues of control are at the root of the problem. In this case both partners should take the essence in conjunction with couples counseling.

There are many sexual problems, diseases and dysfunction that can be treated with Butterflyweed. Some of these include: frigidity, impotence, a number of genital diseases and sexual addictions.

Cats or dogs who develop problems of urinating in the household can benefit from this essence. Animal breeders can use it to increase fertility during breeding time.

Preparation and Dosage: One drop of stock essence per 100 drops of neutral solution for adults, children or animals. For physical symptoms in people, use the stock frequently. Administer three drops 2-3 times per day in a small glass of water.

See Also: Bull Thistle, Blackberry Lily, Motherwort.

*   *   *

When we get out of the glass bottles of our ego,
and when we escape like squirrels turning in the
cages of our personality,
and get into the forest again,
we shall shiver with cold and fright,
but things will happen to us
so that we don't know ourselves.

Cool, unlying life will rush in
and passion will make our bodies taut with power
we shall stamp our feet with new power
and old things will fall down,
we shall laugh, and institutions will curl up like
burnt paper.

—D.H. Lawrence

CANADA THISTLE

Cirsium avense

I am at peace with my family.

This is an herb native to Canada. It grows wild in clumps and has soft pink flowers. It is used herbally as a wash for skin imbalances and for several lung conditions. Native Americans used the root tea as a bowel tonic and de-wormer. The leaf tea is a tonic and a diuretic. It was once used for tuberculosis, dysentery, skin ulcers and poison ivy.

Indications: Harbors family grudges; stimulates family intrigue; gossips; has family secrets; has unresolved family of origin issues; experiences betrayal or abandonment by family members; has trouble with authority; feels misunderstood or persecuted; is unable to trust; has feelings of shame, anger, resentment, jealousy, or self-pity, especially related to family issues; is shy or antisocial.

This essence has to do with one's relationship to family and community. Part of an individual's psyche or personality is constructed by how one identifies oneself as a member of larger groups. The development of this part of the personality begins in the family and can be skewed or retarded when, for one reason or another, the experience of family was essentially negative or painful. In these cases, a person's passage into wholeness and balance requires a reorienting of one's identity in relation to a more healthy group. Canada Thistle helps soften and dislodge hardened beliefs, attitudes and feelings in the personality directed towards some aspect of family or community membership.

Although there are times in one's life when resisting group attitudes is necessary for survival, it often can be that one cannot seem to let go of these attitudes even when they are no longer necessary. To grow mentally, emotionally and spiritually, an individual needs to find a way into healthy groups and be able to express his or her positive nature through the positive roles assumed as part of a

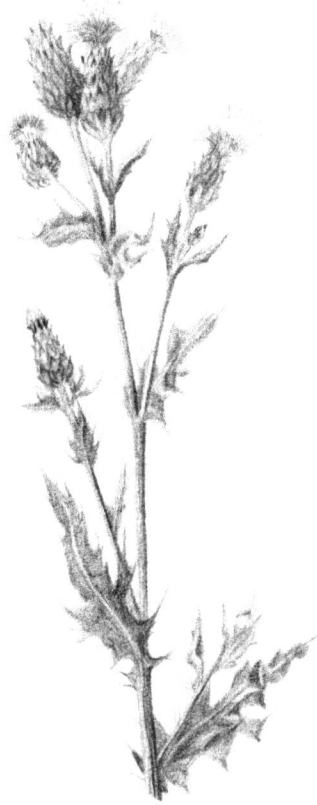

greater whole. Canada Thistle flower essence is a wonderful companion to those who are re-establishing themselves as positive members of strong and healthy families and communities.

Use Canada Thistle for those who are afraid of being with people; for those who have consistent negative reflex response to authority figures; for those who have damaged mental boundaries resulting from indoctrination or brainwashing; for those who are recovering cult victims; for young adults who feel cynical, ambivalent or confused about commitment to having families; for those who have had abusive family lives or who have been betrayed by parents or other role models who were trusted and for those adults who still have unresolved issues with family of origin members.

Canada Thistle is helpful for working with some types of paranoia or feelings that one is being observed or persecuted by government agencies or by clandestine forces. It is also useful for clearing past life imprints of persecution when they signal from the subconscious through dream experiences.

Energetically, higher energies are brought into the deeper subconscious mechanisms of the second chakra. Here are contained the early imprints, which have the greatest influence on our choices and tendencies in all our relations. Stimulating these can make unconscious information regarding our family origins more available to the conscious mind. Processing, release, integration and change are more possible.

This essence should only be used occasionally, and for no longer than two cycles or two months at a time. During this time, it is important that the individual have the space and support to work on those issues that arise during the essence treatment. Psychodrama is a modality that works especially well to complement this essence, or family therapy if the issues in one's present family begin to pattern on family of origin dysfunction. For instance, if one had a violent parent and begins acting with violence to his own children, family therapy would be helpful along with taking this essence.

Use Canada Thistle to help animals who move from small to larger families, or those who may have previously been part of a large family and were mistreated or subjected to over-stressful family living.

Preparation and Dosage: Add one drop of stock essence per 100 drops of neutral solution. Dosage is three drops given twice daily.

See Also: Blackberry Lily, Japanese Knotweed, Motherwort, Blackberry Lily, Comfrey.

CELANDINE

Chelidonium majus

I understand. I am understood.

Celandine is an early spring herb that is seen around many houses and yards. Herbally it is used to treat gall bladder afflictions. The orange sap from the stems is used to remove warts. The signature is quite specific. While the leaves and flowers of the plant grow in a convex fashion symbolizing reception, the seedpods grow upward simulating a transmission antenna. The Latin name for Celandine is *Celidonium* which means "of the swallows." Swallows were observed rubbing Celandine on the eyes of their young to improve their sight.

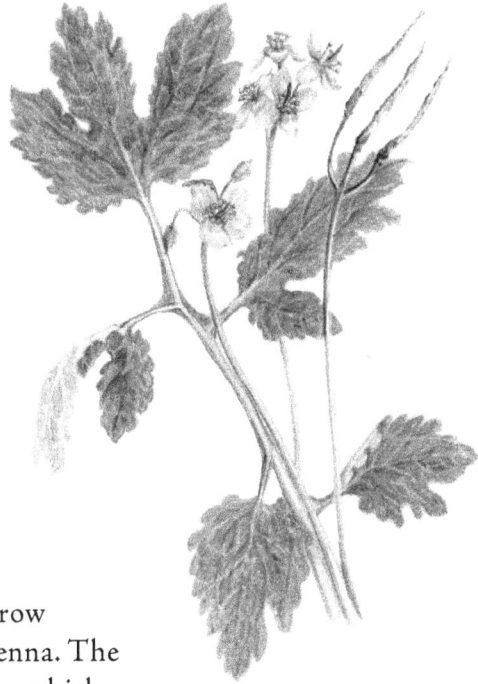

Indications: Has difficulty speaking to others; feels unexpressed; feels misunderstood; has fear of speaking to groups; seems shy; has jaw or throat problems; is quarrelsome or withdrawn; avoids socializing; can't get point across; feels blocked, frustrated; can't receive the message.

This flower essence promotes an enhanced sensitivity to reception and transmission of information. Teachers, lecturers, musicians, actors, artists and writers will find enhancement in their work from Celandine flower essence, as will students and apprentices of any discipline.

Celandine's action is not limited to sensory or intellectual. One can find an enhanced sensitivity to feelings, intentions and orientations of others. This can be useful in negotiation, forecasting, or for therapists and healers of all types.

Use Celandine when there is any breakdown in communication between individuals or factions within a larger group. Therapeutically it can assist in couples and family counseling, conflict resolution and general frustration in any situation where one is not grasping the lesson being presented.

It can also help as a complementary therapy with a number of diseases and imbalances to the throat, tongue, larynx, or jaw, especially when the imbalance appears to be associated with repression of the impulse to speak, a feeling of frustration, of not being heard or understood or with a feeling of not being able to understand another.

Celandine helps those who are spiritually minded develop a feeling of connection in prayer or in communing with higher beings. It can help those who feel frustrated or cut off from such communication and assists in adding clarity to intuitive information which one is receiving.

Energetically, Celandine enhances the strength and flexibility of the throat chakra. Specifically it stimulates this chakra to receive and use energy from both the upper and lower chakras. One understands, knows, feels connected to and shares simultaneously. This eliminates much of the opportunity to short circuit what one realizes through reflexes of doubt or fear.

Celandine enhances animal training, especially in situations where new behaviors are being introduced. Animal communicators will find enhanced success and clarity in receiving information from pets. In these situations, when the pet is also given Celandine, there may be a noticeable enhancement of the pet's "attempts" to communicate. A dog or cat for instance may present the owner with new and unusual behaviors as if they are trying to "say" something.

Use Celandine when one is learning to connect with spirit guides, nature spirits or angels. Those practicing connection to nature spirits will find this plant a useful subject for these exercises.

Preparation and Dosage: Add two drops of the stock essence per 100 drops of neutral solution. Use the stock essence directly for throat problems. Take a few drops of this 2-3 times a day.

See Also: Lobelia.

*   *   *

I have worn this day as a fretting, ill-made garment
Impatient to be rid of it,
And lo, as I drew it off my shoulders,
This jewel caught in my hair

—The Song of a City Pavement to a Broken Flower

COMFREY

Symphytum officinale

I awaken and remember.

Comfrey is an herb that has a strong presence. It has large leaves, which turn downward at the tips, and tubular, bell-like flowers that attract bees. It has a long and prominent history as a cure for bruises, wounds, broken bones, ulcers, sprains and many other conditions where either internal or external tissue has been damaged.

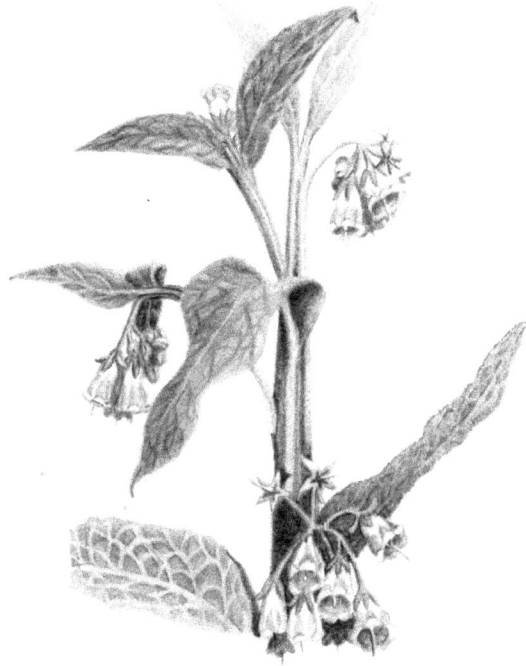

Indications: Is depressed; has a poor memory; has few memories of early childhood; has no memories before age five; can't think clearly about some issues; is anxious; can't remember dreams; can't retain information; tests poorly; has difficulty accessing emotions; is uncoordinated; is restless, anxious, repressed; has irregular heartbeat, high blood pressure.

Just as Comfrey as an herb works to repair tissue and bone damage, Comfrey flower essence provides the same type of repair action on the nervous system. This can have several beneficial effects on memory, coordination, reflex response, biofeedback and restoration of organ functions shut down due to repression.

When memories have been suppressed by the unconscious mind, to protect the psyche from the pain of the event, the nervous system can close down or atrophy around this memory. Comfrey flower essence heals neural pathways that are shutdown, assisting one in gaining access to these memories. With the release of memories, feelings and information to the conscious mind, the individual is able to process and release the pain associated with the experience. In order to have this kind of experience with Comfrey, a person must have done some initial preparatory work in psychotherapy, and have sufficient strength or support to endure the pain of the repressed energies.

General repression — ignoring or distracting oneself from feelings or thoughts that are surfacing — can affect many physiological functions causing sluggishness or imbalance. For instance, unwillingness to allow one's self to feel anger or sadness might slow digestion or cause an irregular heartbeat. Comfrey can, in some cases, ease the stress on these functions. This would occur more in conjunction with a person's wish to relearn healthier emotional patterns of accessing the feelings and expressing them in positive ways.

As the nervous system is the junction between the physical and the non-physical, its stimulation with Comfrey flower essence can increase one's ability to bring information from other levels into conscious awareness. This includes strengthening the ability to recall dreams, deepening meditation and journeying experiences or the developing of channeling abilities.

Energetically, Comfrey works with the deeper layers of the first three chakras, adding energy and rhythm to their functioning. Small movements in these deeper layers can have dramatic and observable effects on the entire psyche. Most repressed information is buried in these deeper layers, while the upper layers contain mostly conscious information. The nervous system is stimulated to receive information from these deeper layers.

Comfrey's powerful awakening action demands understanding and respect. Use it later in the recovery process when a person has learned to recognize and process information arising from the deep subconscious, and has developed a reliable and trustworthy support network.

For animals as well as humans, healing from bone fractures is assisted by Comfrey, as the knitting of the tissues begins with the repair of the nervous system. Use Comfrey also to accelerate healing after surgery. Taking it several times per day starting one week before surgery to several weeks after is recommended.

Prescribe Comfrey for students studying for tests; for athletes seeking better performance in sports, especially where reflex and coordination are key factors in success; for those learning to control autonomic functions such as heart rate and blood pressure; for stressful work and busy schedules when many details must be worked with simultaneously.

Preparation and Dosage: Add one drop of stock essence per 100 drops of neutral solution for most cases where a person is working to relieve patterns of repression. Use one drop per 300 drops of neutral solution when a person is actively involved in awakening repressed memories through psychotherapy, dream-work, hypnotherapy or shamanic journeying. Use the stock essence for treating the physical. Dosage is three drops given three to five times daily.

See Also: Canada Thistle, Milk Thistle, Bull Thistle.

ELECAMPAGNE

Inula helenium

I am beauty.

Elecampagne is a tall plant with large leaves. The daisy-like flowers are a bright yellow. It has been used herbally for a number of lung conditions including pneumonia, whooping cough, asthma and bronchitis. It is also used for stomach problems, to expel worms, as an anti-fungal and as a sedative.

Indications: Fears losing control; fears driving or being in open spaces; feels odd or different from others; feels uncomfortable in social situations; has low self-esteem; is unable to accept compliments; feels unable to change; is cynical; fears driving over bridges; feels misplaced; having identity crisis or mid-life crisis; is socially timid or rebellious; has difficulty identifying with success; has difficulty breathing; is light headed.

Elecampagne flower essence has a strong strengthening and balancing effect on those people who feel odd, different, misplaced or unusual. This can relate to physical attributes, psychological temperament, or a sense of self. A person needing Elecampagne feels estranged from the general population and can have difficulty finding a comfortable identity to work from. There can be either timidity and shyness or a strong expression of personality, which can push others away.

Elecampagne is not for changing a personality, but for making an individual comfortable with his or her own specialness. This comfortability eases much of the social turmoil and aids in the ability to connect with others.

Elecampagne is also valuable in helping those who identify with negative aspects of their personality. In this case learning new traits, skills and behaviors makes no impression on the self-concept. An example of someone who needs this essence, for instance, might be someone who once considered him or herself unintelligent and later continues to have this opinion even when receiving

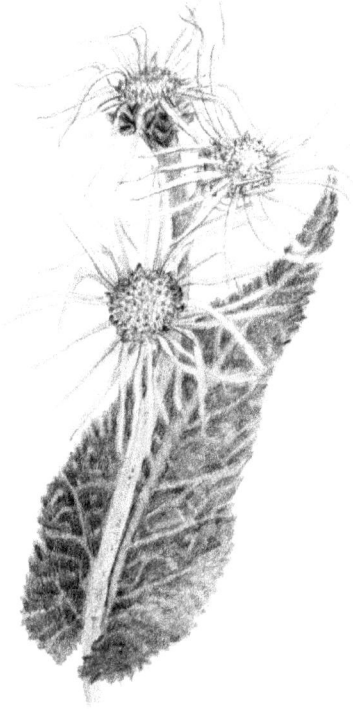

excellent grades in school. Elecampagne helps one transition into a new identity, leaving older more negative imprints behind.

Like many daisies, Elecampagne has its main influence on the third chakra. One fascinating function of the third chakra is to assemble incoming information from other chakras. It is here that one takes the many ideas, experiences, impressions and sensory information and creates a whole or an identity. Without the action of the third chakra, there would be no sense of self. Elecampagne helps this chakra to assemble new information into the energetic structure of the self. Ordinarily, this new information — especially with older people — may be taken in temporarily, but not circulate through the system nor be assembled into the selfhood expressed by the third chakra.

Elecampagne flower essence is an excellent complementary therapy for a number of breathing difficulties in both animals and humans, especially asthma. This is especially true when some of the personality characteristics described above accompany the physical symptom. Elecampagne is also helpful for some forms of agoraphobia or for light-headedness that can occur when a person is driving alone in an automobile.

Elecampagne has broad applications to childhood. It can help with the stress older children feel when a newborn replaces them as the youngest. It can help younger children with the stress of measuring up to standards set by older children. It can also help extreme competition between siblings. It does this by providing a new level of self-acceptance.

This is another essence that is good for animals who have been rescued or who come from abusive previous owners. The personality of the new owner and the safety of the new situation are internalized more quickly. This can have an effect on many physical imbalances that come from projecting old stress onto a new situation. In this case, it is best to give the essence after the animal has been with the new family for at least a few days.

Preparation and Dosage: Add one drop of stock essence per 100 drops of neutral solution. Take stock essence to treat physical symptoms. When treating a fear attack, give this essence at the dosage or stock level once every 15 minutes until the affect of the fear has abated.

See Also: Jack-in-the-pulpit, White Columbine.

FRAXINELLA

Dictamus albus

I evolve constantly.

Fraxinella is also called "gas plant." It emits a flammable gas, which explodes into a burst of blue flame when lit. All of this happens without harming the plant. Herbally it is used as an expectorate and to treat infections, lung problems, and edema.

Indications: Feels stuck; tends to repress feelings or memories; is unable to cope with life; can't seem to change patterns or behaviors; is depressed; has problems with addictions; has had a recent traumatic experience; is cynical; is congested; is prone to inflammations; is frustrated; is obsessed with a past experience; holds grudges.

Fraxinella flower essence helps in many situations and times in our lives when we feel that we cannot get past or resolve an issue. This can include personal issues, issues between partners or group issues that cannot seem to be resolved. Those needing Fraxinella feel more frustrated than helpless. It is as if the energies towards a positive solution themselves cause more discord and misunderstanding. This frustration usually includes both emotional issues and mental attitudes, which can conspire to lock a person into a belief that no relief or change is possible, or to accept a general cynicism about life. Indeed, the basis for these attitudes is one's own experience of difficulty in personal change.

At times we struggle with an issue for so long that it seems to become part of us. Sometimes we continue to struggle without success and other times we simply yield to the belief that we will always have this difficulty. This can be a fear, a habit, a disposition or problem that will not resolve or turn around. Taking Fraxinella helps people to redirect their energies. There may be a short period of inactivity where the psyche begins to withdraw from the frustration

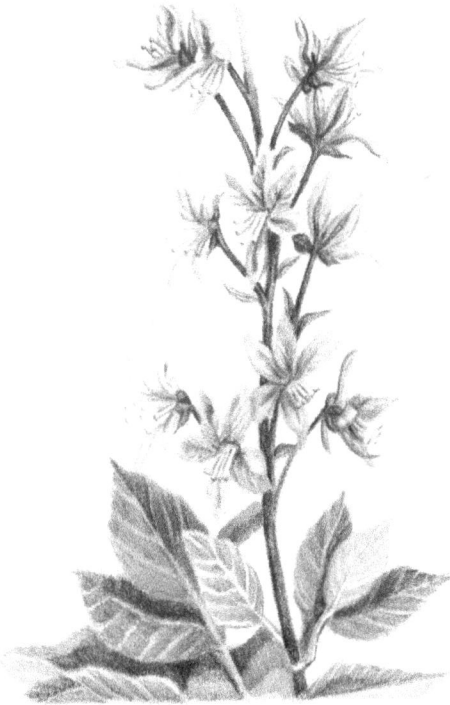

to gain energy. There can, during this time, be a feeling of deep relief as energies of frustration are dislodged and moved out of the energy field.

The fire element of this plant is a key to its energetic action. Fraxinella flower essence will ignite or add a boost to the entire system. Here, lower vibrations that are stuck or heavy will begin to circulate, an ideal situation for creating movement or dealing with buried issues.

Along with the release of frustration often come new ideas and possibilities that have not previously been considered. Often there are flashes of insight or inspiration accessing creative solutions to problems that have been around for some time. Along with these ideas come redirected energies to tackle these problems directly and aggressively. Fraxinella can be especially useful in working groups when frustration replaces more positive feelings towards success.

Fraxinella also helps to ease and heal hurt or trauma that is more recent rather than trauma that has been buried in the past. Incidents of failure, personal tragedy, trauma or misfortune can be eased more quickly with this essence. This is an excellent remedy for short-term psychotherapy for recent victims of violent crimes as it keeps the energies of hurt and pain from sinking into the subconscious.

This is an excellent essence for children who tend to hold grudges or those who are easily frustrated by failure. It can help balance both of these conditions, helping the child stay away from identities and attitudes that might hold the patterns within the personality.

This is a good essence for rabbits and certain other animals who live in confinement, especially when they are prone to cysts, infections and blockages. It is also a good essence for frustrations, which arise when an animal will not respond to training, either in general or related to specific behaviors that an animal may have trouble learning. In this case it is best if both the animal and the trainer take the essence.

Preparation and Dosage: Add one drop of stock essence per 100 drops of neutral solution for most treatments. Use the stock-level essence for treating recent trauma or frustration from a recent event in short-term counseling.

See Also: Horseradish, Habanero Pepper, Milk Thistle.

Golden Amaranthus

Amaranthus hypochondriacus

I move with the flow of life.

Most members of the Amaranthus family grow into beautiful spires, which then begin to droop as the flower matures. The golden variety is one of the lowest and most compact. It was once widely cultivated by the Aztecs who used it as a grain. Corrine Helene, a contemporary herbalist and mystic, describes Golden Amaranthus as the flower which is used to represent victory over death. The signature of the plant is in the way the weight of the blossom bends and directs the plant back to the earth; a lesson in surrender and letting go.

Indications: Is willful; is easily or regularly frustrated; has swings of intense energy and depletion; overworks; is competitive; repeats failures; can't rest; has weakened immune system; is tired; is a perfectionist; is depressed, worried about what might happen, over-committed, generally mistrustful; goes against the tide; succeeds through personal resources; has a number of non-serious health problems; fears fate and sometimes spirituality; is unfocused or unexpressed; takes risks; is original, charismatic, competitive.

Those needing Golden Amaranthus often have great talents, resources and energy and can be moderately to very successful in their endeavors. A hallmark of this personality, however, is a lack of ease or a general sense of frustration with one's self, with others or with life in general. It is sometimes hard to tell with such an individual just where the source of frustration comes from. On one hand the individual may have a strong belief in his own abilities and resources. On the other hand there may be suspicion or mistrust of others. Or there may be an over-reliance on one's self, based on a deep sense of aloneness. In all cases the result is the same: the individual's deep internal struggle, a general sense of separateness and regular frustration.

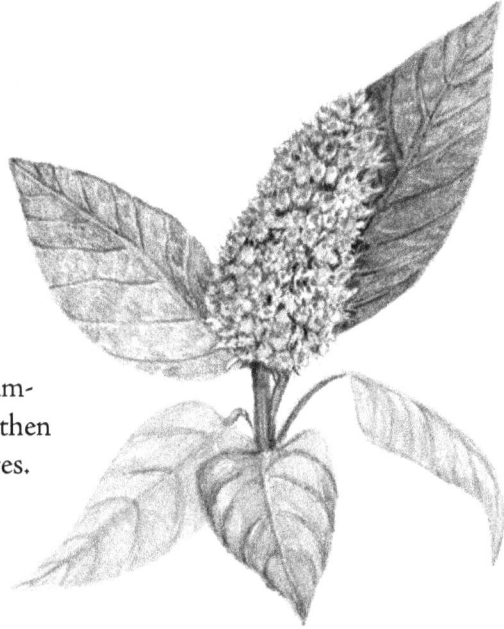

One frustration can be with other people who never seem to be capable enough to deserve the trust needed that would allow the individual to let go and have more time and ease in their lives. Instead, there is a continual disappointment with others who do not perform in a way that meets the standards of this individual who ends up feeling regularly disappointed or betrayed and does the task himself.

Another frustration is with time and events, which seem to conspire constantly against success. There is never enough time and things regularly go wrong. It can feel to this type as if the forces of evil or of good are in conspiracy against him. It can feel as though the individual were fighting against fate itself.

One curse of this personality type is to continue to try and try again even when all outward signs say to stop or to try something else. The over use of will forces eventually can cause breakdowns in both health and relationships. It is as if the spinning of the wheels takes the person deeper and deeper into their own reality where the ideas, feelings and opinions of others mean less and less. This is a classic leadership type who answers the call, takes on the task or responsibility, outperforms the competition, yet privately feels alone, misunderstood, and frustrated about relationships, failures and imperfections.

Golden Amaranthus connects us to the part of the self that "knows" that we are protected and guided on the highest level. It is the connection to this certainty that gives one permission to let the guard down, to trust, to enjoy, to go with the flow, to "let go and let God." In this vibration, health and vitality flourish.

Energetically, Golden Amaranthus connects the three lower chakras, especially chakra three to the sixth. The "knowing" from the sixth is transmitted to the lower chakras. This takes the individual into a bigger picture where control and success are part of a larger reality. The stress of attachment to daily performance and success is eased considerably. The individual can experience setbacks or even failure without obsessive frustrations. Although the essence works more efficiently if the process is conscious, there is still benefit if the individual is unaware as to why he or she feels more relaxation, assurance and ease.

This flower essence is also useful for any personality during times when there are challenges and obstacles that require an intense engagement of our energies, when we have a hard time letting go and relaxing. There may be a waning of energy or a number of small but persistent health problems. It is an ideal essence for students during junior and senior years of high school and college, and for any "fast track" upwardly mobile professional who feels that priorities may need to be reset.

Golden Amaranthus can be effective with animals who have terminal illness.

In some cases, there can be an easing of the symptoms of the disease; in others, there is assistance in making the experience of passing peaceful, dignified and sacred. In many cases, it is useful to prescribe this essence to human family members of an animal who may be close to death but hanging on in spite of many challenging symptoms. Here the animal may be sensing the conscious or unconscious desires of the human companions to have the animal remain in incarnation. Dogs, especially, because of their nature to serve and obey their human masters, can delay their passing because of sensing these desires. Golden Amaranthus assists the transitioning process by helping the family members let go of their own needs and yield to a higher good.

Preparation and Dosage: Add four drops of stock essence per 100 drops of neutral solution. Take a few drops of this 2-3 times a day. Use the stock essence for treating the immune system.

See Also: Blue Vervain, Lemon Balm, Blessed Thistle.

GRAVEL ROOT

Eupatorium purpureum

The Presence of the Divine
is with me always.

A traditional herbal treatment for kidney stones, Gravel Root grows in wet areas and blooms a profusion of reddish flowers in August. A member of the Eupatorium family like Boneset and Hemp Agrimony, Gravel Root grows tall and in spreading colonies that are visible from a distance. Also called Joe Pye Weed, it has been used to treat urinary tract stones, incontinence, impotence, uterine prolapse, asthma and homeopathically to treat gall bladder ailments.

Indications: Fears being alone; fears being in crowds; fears spiritual practices; fears own thoughts; has kidney pains or stones, urinary tract or bladder cysts; is

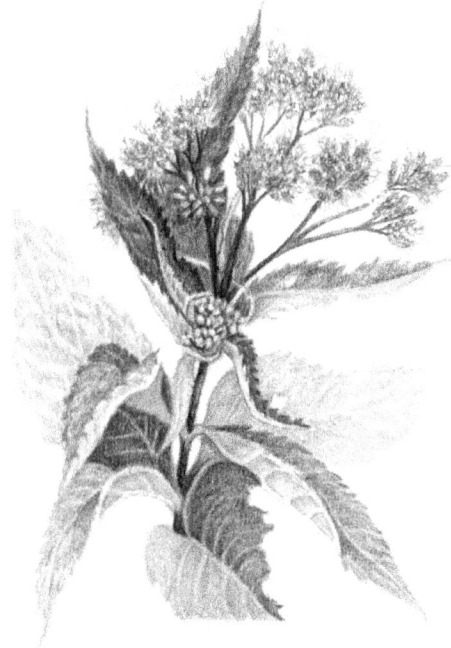

blocked spiritually; has a waning of courage before venturing outward; is anti-social; resists socializing; socially withdraws; is obsessed with own ideas; is angry and disappointed with friends; feels betrayed; feels not accepted by others.

Gravel Root essence treats various types of fears related to aloneness. The first category of these is psychological, for when alone, we meet first the impact of the power of our own thoughts. This can be bothersome, for the mind can take on certain frequencies that are beyond the control of a person and have negative, fearful or destructive qualities. This is especially true when the thinking process has not been guided by wise and loving parents in childhood, or when a traumatic event has altered the natural flow of positive thoughts from the psyche. In these cases there can be a general avoidance of solace and an over-dependence on the stimulation of the mind from the outside. There is a great trend in present cultures to distract the mind with constant and powerful stimulation. Gravel Root flower essence eases this type of fear, allowing a person to gradually accept and benefit from periods of solace.

There are key times in a person's life when one must separate from loved ones or the familiar and venture out on one's own. Starting a new job, going away to college, moving away from a very safe and familiar neighborhood are examples. During these times an individual may feel a deep feeling of aloneness and a corresponding fear. Gravel Root eases the fears associated with these changes, allowing a person to feel a steadiness and confidence.

The underpinnings of these types of fears are very spiritual in nature, for it is when one is alone that one meets God. There are many experiences available in meditation, reflection, retreat and prayer that exceed the realm of the comprehension of the deductive mind. This causes fears, blocks and avoidance of these experiences and those practices that allow them into awareness. In some cases the fear is so buried in the unconscious and so intense, that a denial of the existence of God and higher realms finds roots in the mind and grows into atheism. Gravel Root eases resistance to exploring these states and eases fears of attempting to move forward in spiritual seeking.

Gravel Root can be used to treat general loneliness or a lingering pain of loss of a spouse or close companion. It can treat antisocial tendencies or extreme dependence on other people's company. It is good for artists, musicians or any profession that requires long hours of separation from people. It is a wonderful companion essence for vision quests and spiritual retreats. It is also recommended for herbalists, fishermen, environmentalists, gardeners and naturalists who spend a great deal of time away in nature.

Energetically, Gravel Root enhances the ability of the second chakra to form solid, healthy, conscious connections with others. Primarily this happens through the use of filaments or emanations from the second chakra. We use these to form relationships. Forming healthy conscious relationships protects this area of the system from fears. When the healthy (in this chakra) individual is alone, he or she can access the energy from the connection to others, while the unhealthy individual cannot.

Sometimes individuals who work to develop ideas or projects in isolation from others can become attached or even obsessed with their thinking. This is especially true when there are not good healthy relationships available to anchor the person. This absence of close relationship, coupled with an intense involvement with one's work, can cause the third chakra to increase in velocity, breaking rhythm with the second. This often results in vanity, elitism or ego-ism. It is as if one's thoughts actually replace relationships, becoming grandiose, distorted, obsessive and self-serving. Here Gravel Root, by enhancing the second chakra, rebalances the relationship between the second and third chakras, making distorted thinking less likely.

The types of fear associated with this essence can cause certain vulnerability in the kidneys and the bladder. Gravel Root flower essence, in relieving fearful states and anchors in the psyche, can help with calcifications and cysts in both these areas. Since the vibrational nature of this preparation works directly on the level of the mind and emotions, it will have a cleansing and stimulating effect on the kidneys by relieving fears that cause the physical imbalances.

Cats who have difficulty associating with other family animals or who are generally anti-social or feral, will benefit from this essence. Dogs who are left alone, put outside on guard, or who live outside the family home in a doghouse, will benefit from Gravel Root. Here the essence lowers the stress that results from these situations. Give this essence to any single pet living in a household as a general tonic for increased health and improved temperament.

Preparation and Dosage: For most complaints use a dosage bottle containing two drops of the stock essence per 100 drops of neutral solution. Add five drops of the dosage bottle to a small glass of water and sip over a period of a few minutes. Do this two to three times per day, preferably during short periods of quiet. For most physical problems, add ten drops of the dosage preparation to the water. For painful cysts or stones in the kidneys, take this preparation every hour until some relief is felt.

See Also: Marshmallow, Hemp Agrimony, Pink Amaranthus, Blackberry Lily, Japanese Knotweed.

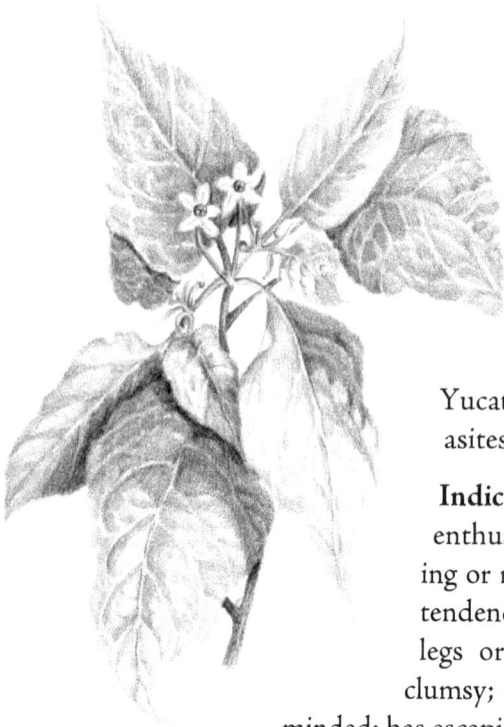

HABANERO PEPPER

C. chinese haberno

I am totally present.

Habanero Pepper is one of the hottest peppers in the world. Native to the Yucatan, it is used herbally as a purgative for parasites and in many dishes requiring a zesty flavor.

Indications: Is lethargic; is unable to feel joy or enthusiasm; is sluggish; has difficulty concentrating or remembering; has lower back problems; has tendency towards poor circulation; has weakness in legs or knees; has vertigo; is depressed, erratic, clumsy; cannot think clearly; daydreams; is absent-minded; has escapist tendencies; has sexual difficulties.

Soul force begins its descent into the physical from conception and birth. As we pass from childhood through adolescence to adulthood, soul energy occupies more and more of the physical. When this happens in a healthy and natural way mental development proceeds normally and the lower organs stay healthy. Trauma at any time causes an interruption in the descent of these energies. Energies of pain and hurt can then take hold in the physical and block the flow of the higher vibrating soul energy. Moreover, if a trauma occurring in childhood is repressed and unattended into adulthood, then physical symptoms can manifest, especially in areas of the body related to the lower chakras: the legs, lower back, circulation, intestines, kidneys and pelvic area.

Habanero Pepper catalyses movement of repressed energies related to trauma to the surface, creating more room for the circulation of soul energies. For this reason Habanero Pepper is an excellent remedy to accompany psychotherapy with trauma survivors.

The heat of this pepper, and the downward shape of the pepper symbolize the action of this essence on the chakras. More rapid velocity in the lower chakras tends to clear lower vibrational "debris" out, making room for more soul energy to enter. The result of this is more "awakeness" or presence, and the potential for movement forward.

It is a helpful essence with vertigo, disorientation, clumsiness, some forms of dizziness, lethargy and depression. It provides stability and balance to "wandering souls," as its main action is both deepening the penetration of soul force into the lower chakras and the alleviation of several forms of mental fogginess.

Very often those needing Habanero pepper will have a strong reaction to holding the bottle of essence. A spontaneous feeling of repulsion can indicate that the person is not yet ready for this essence. Indications for readiness to use this essence include a strong support system of friends and professionals and an ability to process deep and painful feelings.

Children or adults who had any kind of complication, difficulty or trauma in the birthing process and who later develop difficulties such as forgetfulness, absentmindedness or inability to focus, will benefit from Habanero Pepper flower essence.

Use this essence for rescued dogs to change reflex behaviors, which were very likely acquired from previous abusive owners. In these cases, a certain type of voice tone, or behavior — picking up a stick, for instance — may cause the animal to cower or become aggressive. Habanero Pepper, along with certain types of "deprogramming" training will help the reflex to dissipate. In some cases when an animal has a general difficulty in learning new behavior, this essence will prove helpful.

Preparation and Dosage: Add one drop of stock essence to 100 drops of neutral solution for most treatments. Take a few drops of this 2-3 times a day.

See Also: Fraxinella, Horseradish, Lungwort.

*   *   *

I am already given to the power that rules my fate.
And I cling to nothing, so I will have nothing to defend.
I have no thoughts so I will see.
I fear nothing, so I will remember myself.
Detached and at ease,
I will dart past the Eagle to be free.

—*from* THE EAGLE'S GIFT, Carlos Castenada

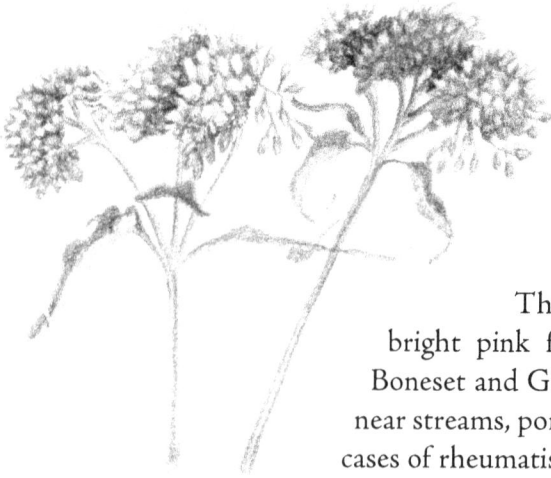

HEMP AGRIMONY

Eupatorium cannabium

I am one with all things.

This plant is tall with reddish stems and bright pink flowers. It is in the same family as Boneset and Gravel Root and thrives in damp places near streams, ponds or bogs. It is used herbally in some cases of rheumatism. It is used as an expectorate, and in larger doses as an emetic and a laxative.

Indications: Feels disconnected; is unable to feel closeness to others; feels alienated or in exile; has many social fears; is reluctant to socialize; is mistrustful or judgmental; is on guard; does not feel "belonging"; is loud or unfriendly; feels disconnected from the earth; fears nature; fears bodily functions; has difficulty feeling "at home."

Hemp Agrimony helps people access and develop the ability to connect to others. Often, those who are judgmental, shy or fearful of social contact are holding on to some imprint: a fear, memory, feelings, etc., which tells them it is unsafe to be with others. There are often feelings of deep ambivalence about socializing. One feels an inclination to connect but also a reluctance that can be conscious or unconscious. Those needing this essence often have partners and families, and appear very social. One clue is that they avoid social engagements and look forward to being alone, but feel something to be missing.

Hemp Agrimony provides two healing actions. The first is the release of the imprint(s) that prevent the feeling of connection. These can be negative experiences in school, damaged friendships, or attitudes of deep mistrust about people, which are either rational or irrational and unexplainable.

The second action of the essence is to assist the individual in opening to a certain spectrum of the love vibration where one begins to understand the meaning of connection to one's self, to the earth, to God, the universe and to others. It is not as if the essence in itself teaches these things, but more that the individual is better able to internalize and act on these realities from a deeper sense of the meaning of "self" as a part of a whole or collective. Working with this vibration is a journey in and of itself. Individuals using this essence can develop strong qualities of compassion, altruism and leadership that were previously not accessed.

Energetically, this essences enables various parts of the chakra system to make connections: the first chakra to the earth, the second to people we choose to be in relationship with, and the crown to connect to higher information. These connections are brought into the system for use and potential integration.

This essence can ease selfishness and extreme independence in children. It can also assist adolescents in the development of leadership qualities and social grace.

Use Hemp Agrimony for animals who are antisocial or very territorial. In some cases, animals who are bred to protect or to be on guard can have difficulty letting down their guard with other animals or humans. Hemp Agrimony helps animals feel their own natural curiosities and connections to others. It can help birds that are very territorial.

Preparation and Dosage: Add one drop of stock essence per 100 drops of neutral solution for most treatments. Take a few drops of this 2-3 times a day.

See Also: Gravel Root, Indian Pipe.

HORSERADISH

Amoracia rusticana

I feel my power.

Horseradish is a white flowering perennial, which is noted and used today for the root, which contains very spicy oils. Horseradish is used to add heat and flavor to many culinary dishes. It is also used herbally to stimulate sweating and to treat asthma, bronchitis and other respiratory ailments.

Indications: Feels stuck; feels unable to make change; feels powerless; feels lethargic; feels controlled by fate or by others; feels

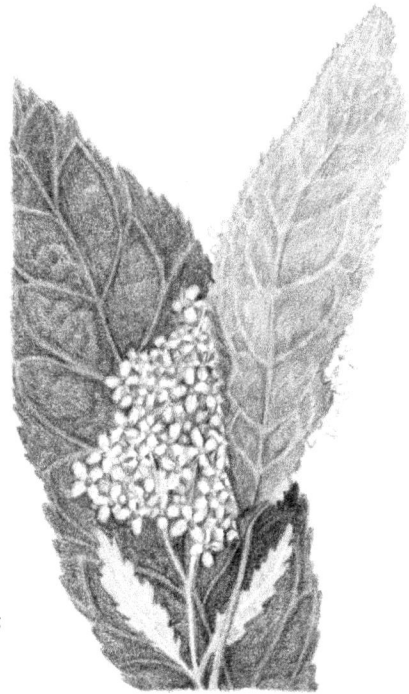

unable to have the life one wants; has low self-esteem, lack of vigor, obsessive thinking patterns; blames others for problems and shortcomings.

The core issue addressed by Horseradish flower essence is a person's feeling of their own power over their world—their ability to change things, to manifest things that they want in their lives. Powerlessness has many levels, many faces and many symptoms, which are addressed by this essence.

Horseradish flower essence is useful in situations where a person feels "stuck," especially when the idea of moving forward evokes a fear that results in inertia. In cases like this, a person often finds ways to avoid facing the real issue and can often throw much energy and action into matters of less significance. In some cases, obsessive thinking patterns can develop, or a depression sets in where one feels separated from one's true self or from one's real mission and goals in life. On the surface and to others the person can seem busy, productive and involved, while inside feelings of helplessness and separation reside.

Horseradish brings the real issues and problems into focus where they can be dealt with: fears are often released and vital energy is made more available for use for important matters. Feelings of frustration and powerlessness are eased and a person is likely to feel more confidence. These subtle shifts often happen imperceptibly over the course of time. But they can also, however, emerge right away. Health, vigor, success, esteem and personal power will all improve.

When taking Horseradish, it is good to have a goal or metaphor of success to work with. Goal-directed energies are enhanced greatly. Small successes can release confidences that were previously trapped by subconscious feelings of fear, inadequacy and powerlessness. These reserves find their way to the surface when horseradish is used to help the individual move forward.

Children who tend to be timid and lack confidence can benefit from this essence. Older children preparing for college and career choices would benefit from this essence, especially when there seems to be avoidance and procrastination over these issues.

Energetically, the third chakra is stimulated to coax an individual to *act*. At first this might feel confusing to the individual but with coaching he or she can feel more able to do things that previously felt impossible. The stimulation of the third chakra also affects confidence.

Use Horseradish flower essence for animals who become depressed and inactive in response to owners feeling or expressing "bad temper" during stressful times. It is helpful for animals who tend to have poor circulation, slow digestion or colds.

Preparation and Dosage: Add one drop of stock essence to 100 drops of neutral solution for most treatments. Use frequently—as much as every two hours —until the person begins to respond. Three drops given three times per day is the dosage for most treatments.

See Also: Fraxinella, Habanero Pepper, Lovage.

HYSSOP

Hyssopus officinalis

I release guilt forever.

Hyssop is a low-growing, blue or white flowering perennial, which is sometimes grown as a hedge or border planting. It is used herbally for sore throats, stomach problems, coughs and poor digestion. It is used externally for burns and inflammations.

Indications: Feels guilty; feels undeserving of happiness; has stomach problems; has problems in food assimilation; has mineral deficiencies; has feelings of foreboding; has fear of punishment; has difficulty enjoying; fears pleasure; feels fear when successful; engages in self-sabotage.

Hyssop flower essence addresses hidden parts of the psyche which one has chosen to keep hidden from others. These include issues of guilt, self-blame, shame and fears of being judged. It might be that these have been transmitted in ways that the person is conscious of, or they might be unconscious imprints from early self-blame or punishment that the individual is unaware of. There are many human dynamics related to these that can be treated with this essence.

For instance, extreme tendencies towards perfectionism are often guilt-based. It is as if one must constantly strive for perfection in order to avoid self-accusation. In this case, the person might be outwardly very successful, but inwardly feels frustration, never feeling the worth of the work being done. The focus is almost always on flaws and shortcomings.

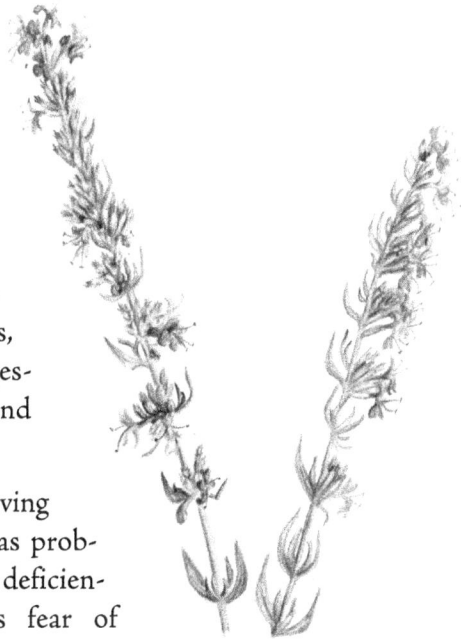

Damage to the self-esteem can be inflicted through blame. Here the individual, in not feeling worthy, refuses to accept nurturing information or experiences, and in doing so keeps the energy from the esteem from being available. Such individuals are unable to accept the very messages that would provide the deep healing which is necessary.

Self-blame is also at the base of tendencies towards judgment of the self and others. Although a certain level of judgment is necessary for protection and self-preservation, guilt-based judgment can be relentless and destructive. Hyssop helps a person "undo" some of the irrational foothold of judgment and self-condemnation, which in turn eases these patterns.

Hyssop is useful for those adults who were brought up in guilt-based families, philosophies or religions. In this case there is an awareness that what has been taught was harmful, but there is still a strong reflex towards guilt when there is a mistake or failure. Hyssop changes one's orientation from blame to acceptance of things as they are. Humanness may be appreciated rather than held in contempt.

Energetically, Hyssop helps to cleanse the second chakra of imprints of guilt, shame and unworthiness. These imprints form a membrane over the chakra, which prevents the person from taking in enjoyment and pleasure. This membrane can also prevent mineral absorption. With Hyssop the membrane loses its density and can begin to move through and out of the system.

Animals who are trained through traditional methods involving physical punishment can benefit from Hyssop, especially in those cases when the punishment is inconsistent and sometimes harsh. It is also beneficial for those animals who are subjected to trainings which are different from the beliefs and personality of the primary owner.

Preparation and Dosage: Add one drop of stock essence per 100 drops of neutral solution for most treatments. For releasing deep guilt patterns, take the essence several times per day for several weeks. After each week, stop the treatment for a day or two and then begin again taking fewer drops of the essence fewer times each week. One may, for instance, begin taking five drops of the essence, five times per day. The second week, four drops, four times, etc.

See Also: Blessed Thistle.

INDIAN PIPE

Momotropa uniflora

I live in the Presence of Love.

This plant has a striking appearance because of its absence of chlorophyll. When picked, the white leaves and stalks turn black. Indian Pipe was once known as "ice plant" because it looks like frozen jelly. Native Americans used the plant juice for inflamed eyes, bunions and warts, and drank the tea for aches and pains due to colds, and as a sedative for pain, restlessness and irritability.

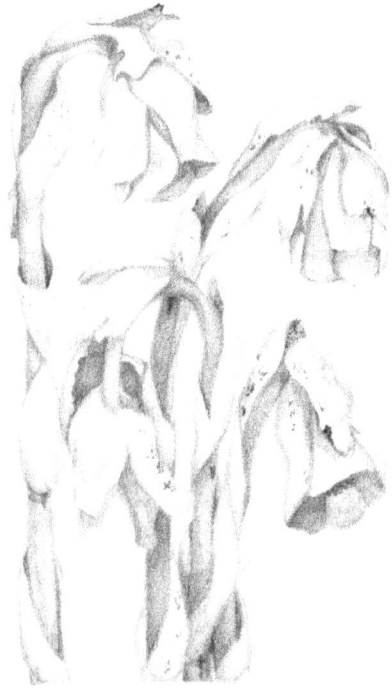

Indications: Feels unloved; feels lonely; is frustrated in relationships; feels disappointed by relationships; seems to need more love; can't understand or accept baser human emotions and actions; can't fight; feels saddened and depressed by many conditions in the world; is a pacifist; can't feel God's presence in the world.

Much of today's world is dominated by a mental stress resulting from intensely busy and challenging schedules. Within this stress, cold efficiency, intolerance and conflict can overshadow love, patience and harmony. Indian pipe is for those heart-oriented beings who have tremendous difficulty relating to the absence of love and warmth in their environment.

Although we know on one level that we were created and are loved by a Higher Being, we tend to feel loved more in some circumstances than in others. Within the arena of life, the presence of a constant Love can become more of an abstraction than a real feeling. Indian Pipe brings this feeling closer and more into focus so that one can enjoy a more constant relationship with a Loving Presence in one's life.

Clinically speaking, feeling the presence of love, however it is received or understood, can heal or ease many afflictions related to grief, loss, separation, loneliness or alienation. Experiencing the benefit of this essence does not require a belief in God so much as an "openness" to the reality of a Presence which one can feel and experience.

Children needing this essence often have loving parents, but must deal regularly with adults or siblings who are not loving or affectionate. Some adults needing this essence may have discovered, sometime in their lives, an experience of profound love, which for one reason or another ends. This may have been a very loving parent or relative, or it may have been a spiritual leader. This can cause a deep affliction in the soul as if "love has gone." Indian pipe brings a feeling of the presence of love causing this affliction to retreat.

Energetically, the crown chakra opens wider to receive higher energies. At the same time all other chakras are harmonized to receive the energy from the crown. A definite sense of "presence" fills the being, and an opportunity to use these energies is available.

This is also an essence for those who are working to develop the vibration of unconditional love in their own beings. Such individuals can falter in this work wondering if the ideal is real or worth the struggle.

Use this essence for those who do not feel loved, children who feel picked on by other children or siblings, children with stern teachers, adults who feel they are in non-loving relationships, animals who change owners, animals who require a lot of affection, pound animals and most caged birds.

Preparation and Dosage: Add one drop of stock essence per 300 drops of neutral solution for most treatments.

See Also: Gravel Root, Hemp Agrimony, Jack-in-the-pulpit.

*   *   *

The talking oak to the ancient spoke,
But any tree will speak to me.
What truths I know I garnered so.
But those who want to talk and tell,
And those who will not listeners be,
Will never hear a syllable
From the lips of any tree.

—Mary Carolyn Davies

INDIAN TOBACCO

Nicotiana rustica

I embrace my higher
nature.

Indian Tobacco, a mem-
ber of the nightshade family,
is a small to medium height
plant with white or yellow
star-shaped flowers. It has
been used herbally for coughs
and throat conditions. It is
used in some sacred ceremo-
nies among several Native
American tribes.

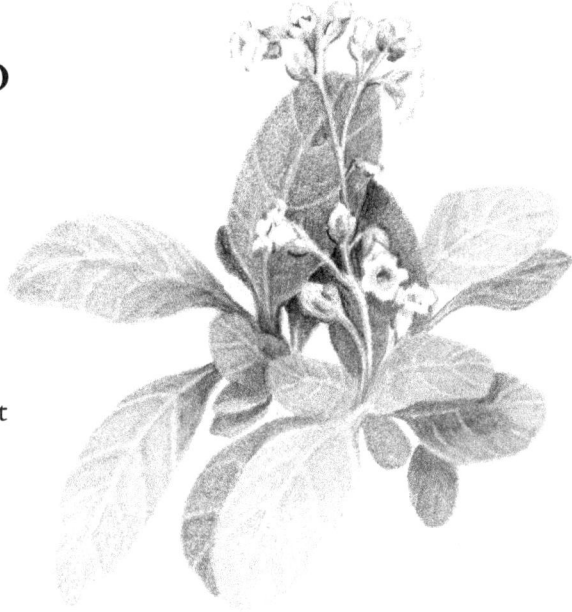

Indications: Fears certain types of spiritual experiences; has difficulty maintaining spiritual practices; fears falling asleep; fears death; is over-rational; is agnostic;
is an atheist, is cynical about spiritual ideas; is materialistic.

Indian Tobacco flower essence helps relieve buried fears regarding one's
relationship to God, to spirituality or to the world beyond the physical. These
fears are largely hidden and in most cases surface only when a person is genuinely seeking authentic spirituality, or has a real and bona fide spiritual experience. In most cultures today the conscious mind is not schooled in the meaning
of spirituality, but rather more deeply imbued in scientific thought and structured religion. These types of thinking do not often give the support to the conscious mind to hold, explain or contain a spiritual experience.

At various thresholds related to spiritual development an individual may feel
the power of an experience, his or her own smallness or lack of control. In all of
these instances, fear can arise causing the person to doubt or retreat from practices, move more deeply into materialism or give up a spiritual quest entirely.

Unfortunately, however, the roots of this fear are often buried in the
unconscious, so the conscious mind may struggle to rationalize reasons for
abandoning the path or practices that have brought up the fear. Indian

Tobacco greatly relieves fears around spiritual experiences or ideas, often bringing to the conscious mind information related to its origin, such as a fear of a parent, a past life initiation or an earlier difficulty with a real spiritual experience. When they are conscious, most fears are more manageable. There is an even, stable reassurance and courage related to spirituality brought into one's being by this flower essence.

Energetically, the first and second chakras release fears, which have been transmitted unconsciously from the sixth chakra. These fears residing in the sixth chakra are from memories of fear or despair related to God and spirituality from other lifetimes. In the lower chakras they become blended with normal human fears, but surface when issues of spirituality come into focus. With Indian Tobacco, the higher influence is better able to reach the lower chakras in an unpolluted form.

This is a good essence for those who are overly cynical about spirituality, those who are overly materialistic and avoid spirituality altogether or those who are indecisive about spiritual direction. It is also helpful for those who are unable to commit to a spiritual path.

Many children have genuine spiritual experiences which they begin to fear or bury when they receive negative feedback or criticism or concern from the adults they share these experiences with, or if they receive negative or fear-based interpretations about what the experience means. In this case Indian Tobacco helps the child to co-exist easily with spiritual gifts or experiences, and not push them into the subconscious because of fear.

Preparation and Dosage: Add one drop of stock essence per 100 drops of neutral solution for most treatments. Use one drop of stock essence per 300 drops of neutral solution for shamanic journeying or past life regression to discover the roots of one's fear of spirituality.

See Also: Black Currant, Jack-in-the-pulpit, Blessed Thistle.

JACK-IN-THE-PULPIT

Arisaema triphyllum

The Divine is within me.

Jack-in-the-pulpit is a woodland
flower that appears in the early spring.
The flowers are green with purple stripes
that fold into a cloak-like configuration over
a tall, yellow anther.

Indications: Is frustrated by religious
thought; is estranged from organized spiritual or religious groups; is spiritually jaded; is
unclear about one's own beliefs; is unwilling to
dialogue; feels abandoned by God; has animosity towards spiritual leaders; is cynical.

This essence forms a vital bridge between incoming spiritual impulses and
one's day-to-day expression of spirituality in the world. The challenge for the
soul in this case is to coordinate what one "feels" to be true with what one has
"learned" is real. Within this dynamic, there can be many difficulties incurred:
feeling unable to express what one feels to be true, self-judgment, inability to
resolve differences one feels between inner feelings and religious beliefs, feeling
judged or misunderstood by a spiritual or religious community.

Jack-in-the-pulpit strengthens one's relationship to the inner voice and
makes more possible the expression of personal spirituality. In this case every-
one benefits. Organized groups and religions receive the benefit of "inspired"
expression, and the individual feels accepted and expressed.

In understanding one's self more deeply and profoundly through use of this
essence, a kind of security and confidence in one's experience begins to grow. A
person is less likely to feel timid and secretive about new ideas and feelings, and
more likely to give expression to them.

This is a good essence for those who have had satisfying religious or spiritual experiences in their past and for some reason have had to leave the group
they were associated with. In this case there can be a feeling of separation from
God or spirituality, as if the connection could only be obtained through one

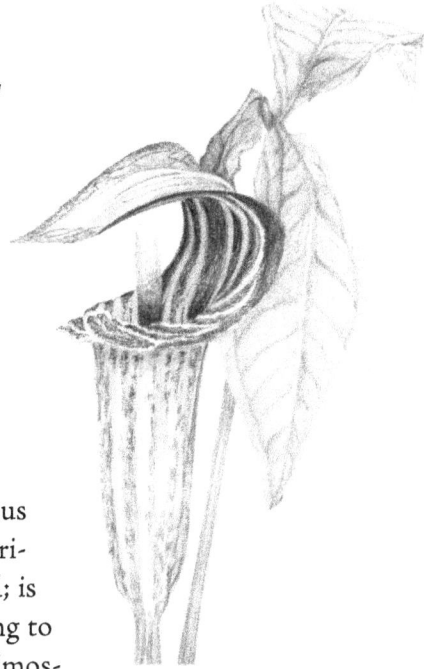

way. Jack-in-the-pulpit teaches the lesson that God is everywhere. It helps bring a feeling of spiritual renewal into the present no matter what the outer circumstances are.

Energetically, higher and lower chakras are bridged. Not only is information from upper chakras brought downward, but the action strengthens the individual to express these truths. There may be a stage of writing or proclaiming that comes about.

This is a wonderful essence for people exploring new forms of spiritual thought, for deep thinkers who feel a frustration, as if they know something but cannot fully express it, or for children who ask many questions about deeper aspects of life and death.

Use this essence for animals who are having difficulty integrating their instincts with their environment. All caged or confined animals who begin to display self-destructive or compulsive behaviors would benefit from this essence. It is a good essence to give to neutered animals, animals who overeat and animals who do not sleep well.

Preparation and Dosage: Add one drop of stock essence to 100 drops of neutral solution for most treatments.

See Also: Pink Lady's Slipper, Lobelia.

JAPANESE KNOTWEED

Polygonum cuspidatum

We are one.

This is a tall-growing, bamboo-like plant which produces lacy, fragrant flowers in the late summer. Although some grow it as a hedge or border, many find it invasive and difficult to remove because of its deep growing taproot that spreads in all directions when the plant is attacked. The tender shoots are astringent and are boiled as a food. It has long been used medicinally in Asia. Japanese Knotweed has a very wide range of actions in the body — enhancing and protecting immune, cardio and nerve function. Recently the roots have been discovered to be a concentrated source of resveratrol. Herbally, it is used in conditions such as heart disease, cancer, HIV/Aids, Lyme's, and neuro-degenerative disorders.

Indications: Feels misunderstood; is unable to function productively in family or in groups; is frustrated by individual group members; has social prejudices; is judgmental; is frustrated with one's membership in a group, family or organization, feels group or family discord; experiences lack of productivity in groups; is not a team player; is new member of group or family; can't accept new group or family member.

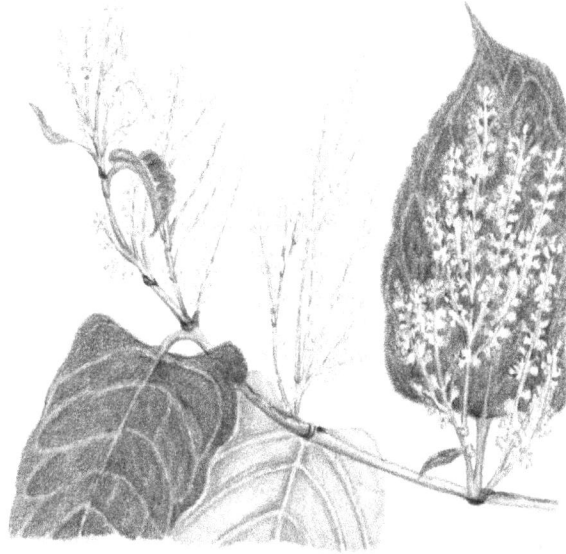

Groups which form today with high spiritual or community ideals often experience a type of frustration, not because of discord in the group, but because of the wide range of differences in ideas and personalities of group members. Groups with divergent energies can have difficulty blending and directing towards a common goal. There can be a feeling of loss of energy, discouragement or frustration because of the amount of time it can take to bring all members to a point of focus or agreement. Japanese Knotweed is a harmonizer of group energy producing a sympathetic bond around all members. Although it is best if all members agree to take this essence before and after meeting, even the presence of the bottle in the room can create a perceivable shift within the group.

Taking Japanese Knotweed to enhance group dynamics can have a number of effects on individual members — not all may experience the same type of vibration from this essence. Some may become quiet while others may feel somewhat stimulated. It is not unusual to observe an increase in humor, agreement, telepathic phenomenon and group efficiency.

For groups already experiencing harmony and efficiency in their business or rituals, Japanese Knotweed can open a deeper awareness that the affairs of the group are being "guided" or assisted by a Higher Power. It can also deepen a "knowing" regarding the correct decision or direction.

Take Japanese Knotweed to resolve any problems or issues regarding goals, direction or differences within any group. This includes couples, families, extended families, living communities, businesses and spiritual groups, especially when there are good relations but differences arise over specific issues or during certain events. Take this essence also to enhance the efficient functioning of any group that comes together for a purpose. Take this essence when new members join a well-established group or when there is a change in membership of any kind.

Energetically, this essence creates rhythm in the chakra systems of group members who use it. All chakras of all members begin to fire in harmony together. This phenomenon takes place naturally among members of an orchestra or singing group when a piece is being played and all members feel part of a single mind or energy.

This essence is helpful for children when a new baby comes into the family. Changes in status and roles happen more smoothly. It is also good when new animals join a family, especially when there are other animals already present in the home. Use this essence also when a new adult joins a family as a partner to another adult who has animals and children who are already bonded. In these cases many growing pains and stresses are relieved — adaptation time is shortened greatly. In each case, best results occur when all family members take the essence.

Preparation and Dosage: Add one drop of stock essence per 100 drops of neutral solution for most treatments. Use as a spray in group areas or meeting places.

See Also: Hemp Agrimony, Gravel Root, Marshmallow.

LADY'S MANTLE

Alchemila vulgaris

"I am masculine. I am feminine."

A strikingly lovely low-growing plant with broad horizontal leaves which expel and hold large droplets of water, and small yellow star-shaped flowers. It has been used herbally to heal damp and congested areas, and more recently as a remedy to help retain firmness in sagging muscle tissue.

Indications: Complains regularly; feels victimized; can't feel one's self apart from others; is over dependent or overly independent; feels unprotected; fears being exposed; feels envious of others; has a slumping posture; apologizes frequently; blames self for others' problems; has blocked creativity; feels scattered or confused; fears leaving home; feels helpless; feels unexpressed; feels insecure; feels uncertain about identity or career; is frustrated, agitated or restless; feels dissatisfaction; has anger attacks; indulges in private feelings of self-pity; reluctant to engage with others; does not feel confident; can be anemic; feels weak; has poor muscle tone; is egotistical and insecure; can't feel feelings; is insensitive; lacks compassion.

In a healthy, balanced personality, both masculine and feminine energies are able to be accessed, circulated and expressed. These are not terms that are conventionally used to express health and balance, but rather are used to describe attributes of the separate sexes individually. Masculine, for instance, is traditionally used to describe attributes of outward strength, harshness and dominance, while the term feminine is often relegated to motherhood, softness and refinement. Energetically, however, this is not exactly the case.

In each person, no matter the gender, masculine and feminine energies work together as a texture of the personality. For instance, creativity, which is assumed to be a feminine quality, has both masculine and feminine aspects. The conception of a creative thought, that is the reception and containment of the inspired information, is the work of feminine energies, while the expression of the idea into form is the domain of the masculine. The creative process includes both functions; the process cannot be complete without the presence and activation of both energies.

What we observe as being masculine and feminine in the personality are often the imbalanced states of these two forces. Dominance, bravado and the show of force, for instance are masculine-feminine energies out of balance. The balanced personality is empathetic, but self-aware; sensitive but secure; risk-taking but cautious; self-serving but generous; ambitious but able to celebrate others' victories; is creative and practical; has a strength that respects its own

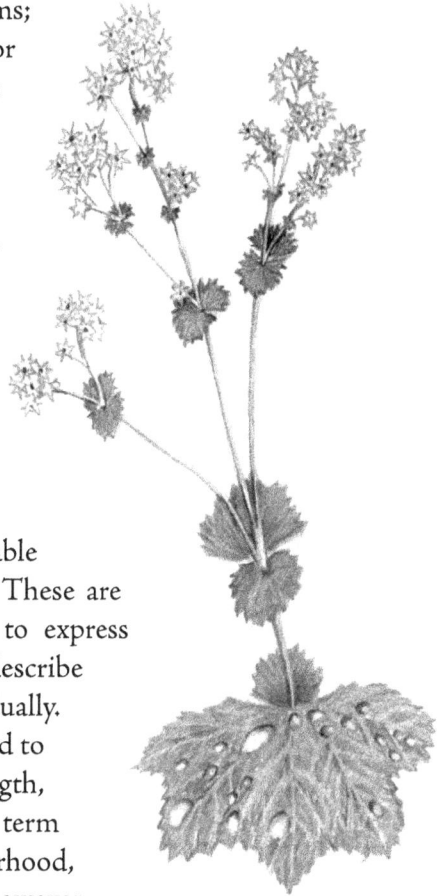

limitations; nurtures others and takes care of self. When we refer to health and balance in the personality, we are really referring to the presence of these forces and the individual's ability to use them.

The feminine aspect of the personality needs a level of safety, respect and recognition through childhood in order to fully develop. It is a more recessive part of the personality which needs the right conditions to gain a foothold in the psyche. The development of the feminine in the personality is made consummately more difficult in a childhood or in cultures where respect for the value of the women or these feminine aspects are not held in respect and importance. For both men and women there are imbalances or adaptations in the personality that has not learned the true value and presence of the feminine. A culture seeped in ruthless competition, resolving problems by overpowering the opposition, learning to dislike others who are different, for example, is a culture ruled by out of balance masculine-feminine energy.

Lady's Mantle is an essence that strengthens an individual's ability to contain and to use masculine and feminine energies in balance. In most cases, this will mean that the feminine aspects that were not cultivated will come more into play, but for each individual, this will mean something different. An aggressive personality, for instance, may sensitize, while a softer personality might gain a more expressive strength.

Energetically, both chakras two and three are strengthened, and the relationship between them is enhanced. Chakra two is attached to the emotional body and chakra three is attached to the mental. These two chakras are designed to work together as a team. With this essence, energy is better able to flow between these two centers without the constant domination of one over the other. A weakness in either chakra will be eased. An unconfident person will feel more strength; an insensitive or unemotional person, more feeling and connection to others.

A second energetic benefit comes about by the stabilizing of the exchange between chakras two and three. The emotional and mental bodies, which are attached to chakras two and three, strengthen so there is less leakage of one into the other. The result is better emotional and mental clarity. The entire protective field responds by contracting slightly; this contraction is beneficial for supporting the healing torn or sagging tissue in the physical, and for strength in the nervous system and the muscles. The slight contraction of the field also helps a person feel more safe, secure and stable.

As its Latin name, *"Alchemila"* infers, this essence can have general and universal uses. There are dozens of applications for this essence and many ways that the personality responds. One can treat both lack of confidence and over confidence; feelings of helplessness, powerlessness, insensitivity, doubt, insecurity, uncertainty and alienation. It is excellent for women who are regaining a lost sense of self, or men who are having identity or mid-life crises. It is excellent for spiritual development or expression of creativity.

Use this essence for women who are taking new risks in their lives, for men who are motivated to improve relationships, and for children beginning to socialize; it is a good remedy for the oldest boy or girl in the family; use it to treat overly aggressive or antisocial animals and pets immediately after being neutered.

Preparation and Dosage: Add one drop of the stock essence per 100 drops of neutral solution for most treatments. When treating clients who had sagging tissue or water retention along with the issues mentioned here, use the stock level of the essence.

See Also: Motherwort, Marshmallow, Golden Amaranthus, Blue Vervain, Borage.

LEMON BALM

Melissa officinalis

I am peace.

Also called Melissa or Balm, Lemon Balm is an excellent herb for the nervous system. It is cleansing, astringent, uplifting, an antidepressant, and has anxiety relieving properties. It is also an effective anti-viral herb. Lemon Balm is a flavorful tea and relaxing in a bath.

Indications: Can't relax; is high strung, hyped up or stressed; experiences mental turbulence; feels on guard; has stomach problems; has tense muscles; feels fears related to resting; feels blocked; feels no inspiration; has writer's block; can't focus; is unimaginative; has performance fears; experiences headaches, insomnia, anxiety.

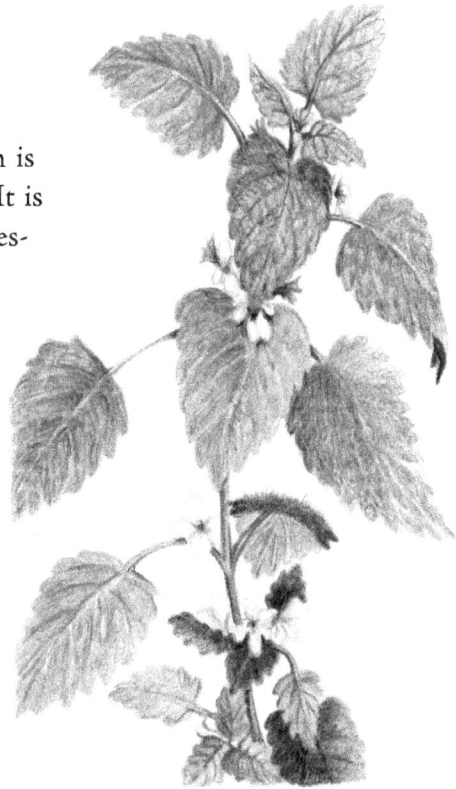

For many people today, for one reason or another, the rhythms of thinking and resting are out of balance. Some have a hard time relaxing because of turbulence in the conscious or unconscious mind. There may be conscious worry or fear over something present and obvious, or there may be some anxiety over something that is less known. Lemon Balm helps the individual rebalance the "breathing" of the activity and rest of the conscious mind and of the unconscious mind.

Lemon Balm's calming action has several beneficial actions. The calmness of the mind, in itself is a state that many today have difficulty with. Calming the mind is necessary for rest, for easing fears and anxieties. A calm mind is necessary in providing protection against stress and breakdowns that the system can experience when overloaded. Lemon Balm provides the means for simple, natural and deep relaxation. It does this by easing the velocity of the mind, which can be agitated by fears that reside in the subconscious. These fears provide a kind of restlessness or hyper-vigilance—the mind is always active. Lemon Balm eases the fears and therefore the intensity of the mind. This provides the opportunity for true relaxation.

At times during the cycle that one takes this essence, there can be the release of fears. This usually happens during the sleep cycle through dreams or through the semi-conscious during a brief period of slight anxiety. These symptoms usually happen in the second or third week of taking the essence. General improved relaxation and sleep often result.

When the conscious mind is eased or resting, other levels of the mind can become active and express themselves. In the dream state we experience this phenomenon. We relax the body and conscious mind and an active state of dreaming begins. The stimulation of the conscious mind ends the dreaming and the body and mind are active once again. The creative processes are another example. These faculties can be enhanced using this essence.

There are times in one's emotional, psychological or spiritual development when there is resistance to what one is experiencing or discovering. This can be information from the past that has been repressed, or it can be past life information surfacing, or higher guidance which one is resisting hearing. During these times Lemon Balm helps move tension and anxiety out so that the needed information can reach the conscious mind.

Energetically, the first three chakras are synchronized to create a downward motion towards the earth. The system naturally does this when a person feels safe and happy. This motion eases turbulence in the mental body, connecting to the third chakra. The mind is now free to receive creative thoughts and inspiration.

This essence is useful with children who are unable to relax or slow down or those who become tired easily. It is useful for the early adolescent stage when a child is beginning to feel anxious about the future. It is useful for stressful periods and for interruptions in the normal sleep cycle. In taking this essence to enhance sleep, it is beneficial to journal one's dream activities to allow unconscious stresses to surface.

Lemon Balm is useful for animals during periods when they are restless and sleep less. It is also helpful to use this essence after an animal experiences an incident of high stress requiring the release of adrenalin. Show dogs and horses will benefit from a single dosage both before and after their performance.

Preparation and Dosage: Add one drop of stock essence per 100 drops of neutral solution for most treatments. Add one drop of stock per 300 drops of neutral solution to enhance dreaming and creativity.

See Also: Skullcap.

LILAC

Syringa vulgaris

I give and receive.

Lilac is a popular bush or small tree that is grown for its showy and sweet-smelling flowers. It is used herbally for insect stings. It is one of the few fragrant plants that resists being condensed into an essential oil but the infused flower oil is used to open the chakra centers.

Indications: Is overly independent; is unable to trust others; is extremely dependent on a few people; has back problems; is a perfectionist; can't delegate work to others; is overly demanding of self and others; is rigid; resists changing plans or standards; has weak lower spine; is easily frustrated.

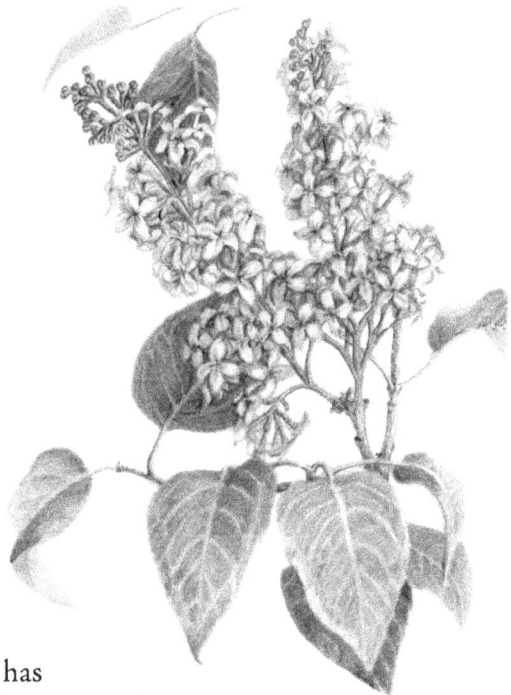

There is a saying that "God helps those who help themselves." Lilac flower essence helps those who will not let others help them. Lilac is for those of us who have learned to over-rely on our own resources and have difficulty in either asking others for help or even in accepting help that is offered. This can mean either very high standards, or a low esteem that does not feel comfortable or worthy to receive assistance from others. It is often the case that a person needing Lilac has fallen into a cycle where s/he set standards too high to achieve and thus sets up a cycle of lessening self-esteem through failure. Next the person overcompensates for the wounded esteem by setting goals that are too risky or too high to achieve. Lilac flower essence helps the person out of these imbalances and assists in developing qualities of true, balanced self-reliance and reliance on others.

Lilac flower essence also helps to heal unhealthy attitudes that often accompany behaviors of extreme self-reliance. These include elitism, perfectionism, a general mistrust of others' ability to perform, a belief in aloneness and separation.

As is sometimes the case with herbs and flower essences, Lilac has an effect on balancing the opposite type of behavior and attitude. Lilac is helpful for those who lean on others too much, not trusting themselves nor willing to hold their own burdens. Often these individuals have unconsciously built a network of friends and acquaintances that are willing to be used in this fashion. In this case Lilac helps a person shift to a feeling of more self-reliance.

Those needing Lilac often suffer from back or shoulder problems, and can have a general "slump" to the overall posture or inflexibility in the spine that causes discomfort. Although these issues can have physical origins, it is often the case that the symptoms accompany a Lilac temperament.

Energetically, the downward pull of the first chakra is strengthened as well as the upward influence of the upper chakras. Here stability, confidence and a sense of self are all enhanced.

Lilac flower essence is good for overly independent or responsible children, or those who seem to fear accepting responsibility. It is good for adolescents who have poor posture and low confidence. It is good for adults who were required to take on adult-like responsibilities very early. It can help a general attitude of apparent "laziness," especially when fear or a lack of confidence causes this. It is a good essence for many types of dogs who feel a responsibility to protect or to perform. In this case it can promote better relaxation.

Preparation and Dosage: Add one drop of stock essence per 100 drops of neutral solution for most treatments. Use the stock-level essence for treating cases where there are spine problems accompanying the emotional difficulties.

See Also: Marshmallow, Motherwort.

LOBELIA

Lobelia siphilitica

I speak my truth.

Blue Lobelia is a medium height perennial herb with spires of deep blue flowers that appear in the late summer. It is used herbally in larger doses as an emetic (its folk name is puke weed), and in smaller doses to treat lung illnesses such as asthma — and for throat problems. Certain Native American tribes used Lobelia for venereal disease.

Indications: Is uncertain about one's own ideas or opinions; is unclear about goals; is uncertain about what one wants; has a tendency towards telling lies; keeps silent in groups; has repressed emotions; is uncertain what to say; feels that words are inadequate; feels insincere; relies on humor; feels inauthentic; cannot say what one wants; hides the truth about one's self; has throat or thyroid problems; speaks softly; is a late talker.

Speaking the truth has many consequences. One can be praised or punished for speaking what one feels to be true. When socialization or family values tend to be strict, harsh or inflexible, it is not unusual for individuals who do not internally align with the conscious values of the group, to "go underground" with their truths, and become publicly silent.

This can mean ideas, philosophies, opinions, feelings, interests, sexual orientations, etc., need to be suppressed. When an individual is not able to fully express inner realities because of fear of shame, punishment, loss of love, etc., then the real impulses retreat deeper into the psyche, and the real personality remains unformed and unexpressed in the world. Although the religious and social fabric today have become more flexible and tolerant of many different types of lifestyles and thinking, still today many situations exist where the real personality remains hidden and unexpressed.

When feelings and ideas are repressed for any reason, over a period of time, a person is likely to lose touch with the feelings. One may not, for example, feel anger or sadness, even when it is healthy and appropriate to do so. Blue Lobelia

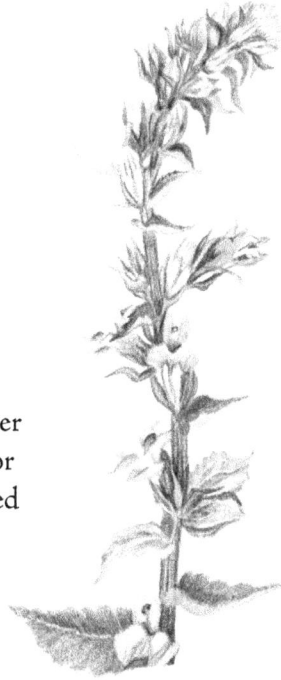

helps one re-sensitize to feelings or other realities, which may be lost. This makes it an important remedy for some stages of psychotherapy. It also helps people who are confused or not clear about their feelings.

Energetically, Blue Lobelia strengthens the throat chakra. This makes it easier for people to speak up about how they feel, what they think, who they are, etc. It is an ideal essence for those who are shy, secretive or unassertive, or for those who feel that it is time to be truthful or "come out" about who they really are. The blue color of the flower expresses not only its alignment with the throat chakra, but also the blue downward channel between the chakras. It is this channel that is activated when a person feels safe. It is as if the essence signals that it is safe to speak.

Lobelia flower essence can be helpful for singers, lecturers and teachers; students who are learning about public speaking, or small children who mumble, speak softly or will not speak at all. It is excellent for children who are late talkers or those who have a problem with stuttering, especially if it is stress related.

Animals that have been punished for being noisy will benefit from this essence. In this case it provides a release of the stress from repressing an otherwise natural instinct. You may also use this when an animal seems to be attempting to communicate something new. This is sometimes the case when new behaviors appear for no apparent reason.

Preparation and Dosage: Add one drop of stock essence per 100 drops of neutral solution for most treatments. This essence may be used externally on the throat or be mixed in a glass of water and sipped. Add one drop of stock essence per 200 drops of neutral solution for treating animals.

See Also: Celandine.

*   *   *

When they have deeply quaffed
From the brimming cups of dew;
You can hear their golden laughter
All the garden through.

—Clinton Scotlard

LOVAGE

Levisticum officinale

I go forward in confidence
and joy.

This plant is a tall perennial with
yellow flowers. The whole plant
emits a strong aroma, somewhat
like celery. The root and sometimes the leaves are used in
medicinal preparations. It is a
diuretic and therefore good for
water retention and urinary difficulties. Lovage is also used for
skin and stomach problems.

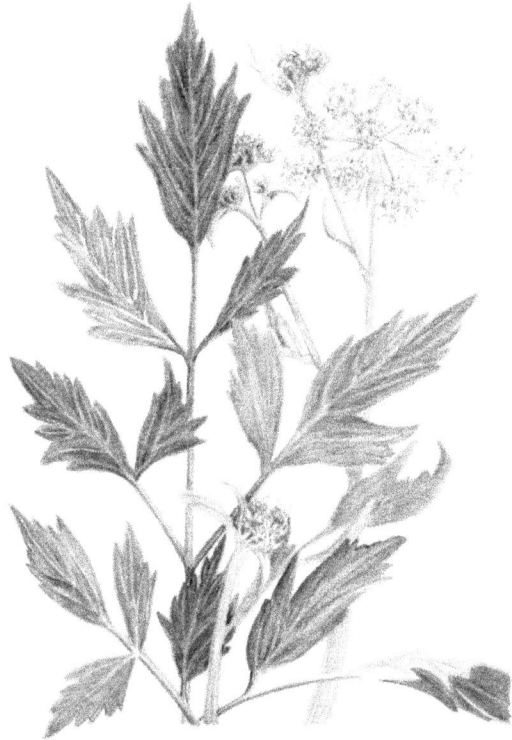

Indications: Is unable to enjoy work; procrastinates; feels stuck; can't manifest
plans into action; is constantly rethinking plans; is fearful about risk; is overly
critical; is an observer of one's own life; is frustrated about one's life direction;
has tendency towards respiratory problems; is afraid to take action; feels
unsafe; has low confidence; feels heavy or lethargic.

Lovage flower essence addresses the dynamic of "doing" or "acting." It helps
an individual maintain a constant momentum of creating or making change in a
positive direction. This is a natural part of the growth process—to be constantly assessing, thinking, feeling, and following through with a structured or
unstructured plan of action.

It is not unusual today for this process to be interrupted—for a person
to become fearful of taking action, too comfortable in their present circumstance, and not allow the thinking and feeling process to catalyze into
action. When this happens, a person "withdraws" from the more fiery energies of action. He becomes less a participant and more of a thinker, talker,
critic or observer of life. The vibration that Lovage flower essence carries is
similar to a combination of strength and joy — the kind of strength and joy
that one feels when life is moving in the right direction. The elation and

solidity come from a feeling of "being-in" one's life rather that being an observer or a judge.

For this reason it is an excellent remedy for those who feel frustrated, disconnected or unhappy about their situations or the direction their lives are moving in, or for those who no longer feel that their lives are "going anywhere."

Lovage flower essence is ideal for those who want to make changes in their lives or want to reconsider redirecting their energies. This may mean ending a relationship or a job that has been unsatisfying for some time, or it may mean starting something new. It may mean continuing forward on one's present course, or it may mean changing directions completely. In any of these cases Lovage adds a level of certainty and confidence that is invaluable for such exploration. Indeed a person can remain in the "in-between" stage, moving in and out of certainty. Use Lovage flower essence to help a person move from the thinking and talking phase to the action phase of making change.

Energetically, Lovage enhances the third chakra to produce a smooth rhythm of energy output. Will forces emanating from this chakra are strengthened. A person therefore has a tendency then to do more; to harness thought energy into action.

Lovage is helpful for children when they begin school, change schools or move to a new home. It is helpful for any stage of life exploration when one considers choices and the future. College selection during junior and senior year of high school exemplifies this.

It is also helpful for more docile or timid animals or those low in the pecking order. It gives an added feeling of contentment, security and strength. It is a good essence to give to dogs that have more than one primary caretaker, when there are strong differences in the style of care, training and discipline they apply. In this case the essence lessens the stress and confusion that is natural to this type of situation.

Preparation and Dosage: Add one drop of stock essence per 100 drops of neutral solution for most treatments.

See Also: Horseradish.

*   *   *

> And 'tis my faith that every flower
> Enjoys the air it breathes.
> — Wordsworth

LUNGWORT

Pulmonaria officinalis

I receive the breath of life.

Lungwort is a low-growing herb with spotted leaves and pink flowers that open in the early spring. The pink flowers turn blue a few days later. Lungwort has been used to treat a number of different lung conditions. It first softens tissue, then cleanses, and then seals or tightens.

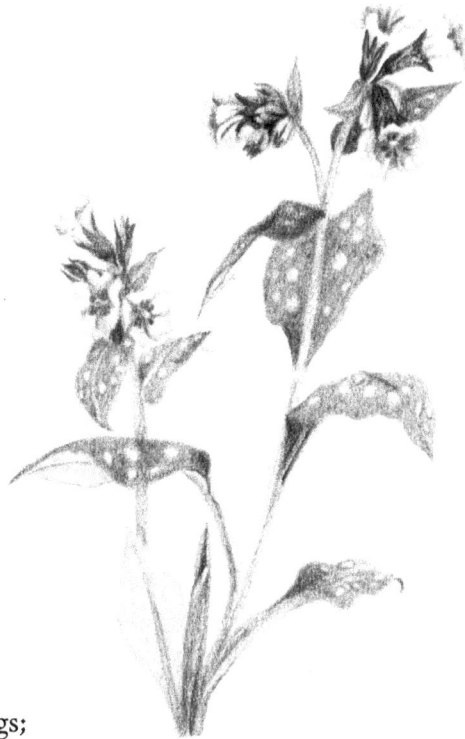

Indications: Feels blocked; breathes shallowly; cannot express some feelings; is afraid of anger; has lung problems; smokes; experiences shortness of breath; has headaches; has heart problems; has stomach problems; is annoyed by small things; can't feel some emotions; has ulcers; has difficulty controlling feelings.

Lungwort assists the chakra system in moving and distributing energy throughout the system in co-ordination with the breathing process. Although the breathing process is an entirely natural process, it can become uncoordinated, inefficient, even dysfunctional over time due to a tendency to not express thoughts and feelings, due to repressed pain in the unconscious, or due to stressful conditions in one's life.

Most often problems in breathing and energy dispersion are manifest as blockages. These blockages are responsible for many physical, mental and emotional conditions. Some examples are: ulcers, heart problems, headaches, obsessive thinking, dissociation or emotional intensification. Lungwort helps to move these blockages out of the system so that energy flows properly in rhythm with the breath. Consequently the abatement of many symptoms caused or intensified by these blockages can be observed.

This concept of moving energy with the breath is the philosophy behind many modalities today, such as yoga, rebirthing, transformational breath or bioenergetics. Lungwort is a wonderful complement to these and other modalities, which use the breathing to move or process repressed energies.

Lungwort can also be useful for many types of breathing difficulties, especially when there is some emotional counterpart to the physical symptoms. Shallow breathing, shortness of breath and asthma are some examples.

When taking Lungwort one becomes very aware of the breathing process, and indeed, it is this added awareness to an otherwise unconscious process that makes lungwort such a powerful complement to breathing therapies. Being conscious of the breath adds strength and stamina to the entire physical system. Use it for those who lose their breath in anxious moments. It is also a useful essence for timid animals and for very shy or sensitive children.

Preparation and Dosage: Add one drop of stock essence per 100 drops of neutral solution for most treatments. Although Lungwort flower essence can be taken internally, it is sometimes more useful to spray it into the air with a mister or through a humidifier. Add 10 drops of stock per quart of pure water. Change the water and add essences at least daily.

See Also: Scarlet Pimpernel, Onion, Milk Thistle, Wormwood.

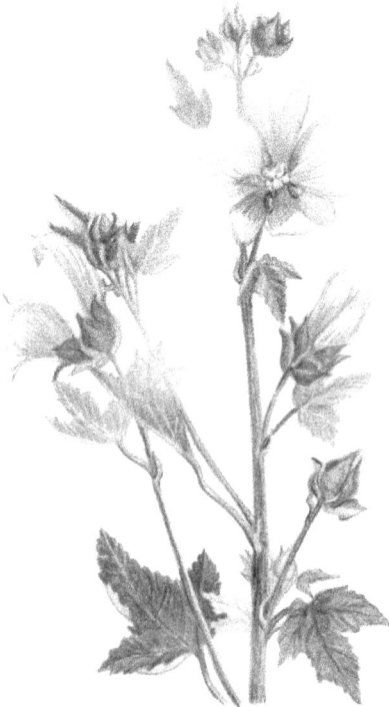

MARSHMALLOW

Althaea officinalis

I allow all to be.

This garden herb is the original source of the marshmallow confection that was made from a gummy substance obtained from the root when boiled. Marshmallow is used to treat kidney problems. It is used, also, as a tea for sore throats and an expectorant for bronchitis. It is applied externally as a poultice for bruises, sprains, muscle aches and inflammations.

Indications: Is inflexible; holds grudges; refuses to listen; won't compromise; is intolerant; is narrow; is antisocial; is hard hearted; angers quickly; has heart problems; can't let go; obsesses about the past; has strong social boundaries; has hardened arteries; is cynical; resolves relationship issues by ending them; can't feel emotions; is rigid.

One reaction to stress today is to toughen or harden as a way of protecting from harm. This may include hardening the conscience against the feeling of responsibility that comes when hearing about injustice in the world; a hardening of the emotions to protect against hurt. Although the response is a natural and a healthy one in itself, hardening as a habit or lifestyle can have many negative effects on the body, mind and emotions. Health and vitality flourish when there is flexibility, versatility, and receptivity in the system.

Marshmallow flower essence helps a person relearn the strength and value of softness. Children, for instance, are naturally able to feel things intensely, and consequently are able to move out of difficult emotional states very quickly. The ability to feel and then let go is an emotional resilience that many adults have lost. Where an adult might stay angry for long periods of time, a child is able to get over the feeling very quickly. Marshmallow helps soften the entire emotional system so that emotions are accessed, expressed, released and forgotten in a shorter period of time.

When prescribing Marshmallow to increase access to feelings and resilience of feeling life, it is important that a person be ready for such changes in the personality. This means having support for changes which can occur, including training and coaching for processing feelings as well as having a system of supportive friends and professionals who understand how to deal with new feelings which are making their way into consciousness.

Marshmallow strengthens the ability of the second or relationship chakra to receive impulses from the heart, and the ability of the heart to send impulses to the lower three chakras. Over one's lifetime the heart chakra struggles to maintain its connection with the lower chakras, and to assert its higher sovereignty over the lower nature. When one chooses hate over love, the lower chakras abrogate their connection to the heart chakra. The heart then loses its ability to function properly within the system. Marshmallow enhances the ability to choose higher emotional values, and supports the functioning of the heart chakra.

Prescribe Marshmallow for emotionally repressed individuals, those who have difficulty in letting go of past hurts, those who hold grudges, and those who fear anger or sadness. Individuals in 12-step programs who are working on accessing their feelings would enjoy this essence, as would children who tend to have difficulty letting go of hurt, anger or criticism.

Marshmallow is helpful for treating any hardening of tissue in animals. It is also a useful complement to retraining animals to be less structured or on guard, or when you are trying to break any previous excessive conditioning. This includes "retired" animals such as show animals, police dogs, racehorses or greyhounds. Marshmallow helps these animals relax and attune to new, less rigid trainers or masters.

Preparation and Dosage: Add one drop of stock essence per 100 drops of neutral solution for most treatments. Add one drop of stock essence per 200 drops of neutral solution for treating animals.

See Also: Motherwort, Milk Thistle.

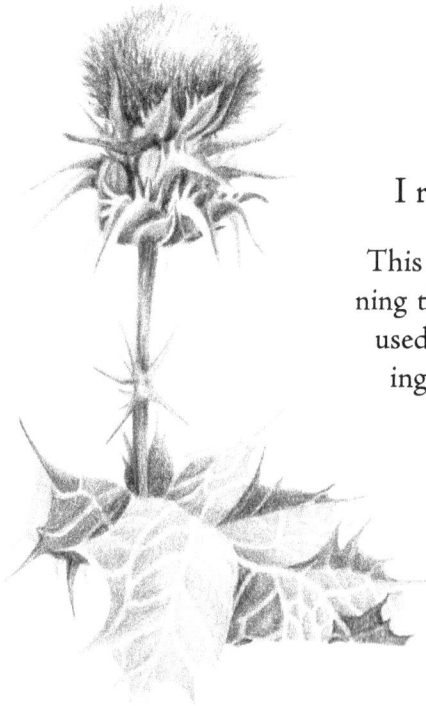

MILK THISTLE

Carduus marianus

I release all that blocks the flow of love.

This thistle is distinguished by the white color running through the green in the leaves. The seeds are used for jaundice, hepatitis, cirrhosis, liver poisoning from chemicals. The herb also dramatically improves liver regeneration when there is disease or poisoning.

Indications: Has an angry personality; can't forgive; has liver imbalances; is a survivor of child abuse; feels unsafe with people; attracts antipathy; dislikes siblings; feels taken advantage of; has gall bladder problems; can't feel or express anger; has elevated liver enzymes; has high blood pressure or heart problems; is prone to inflammations; fears anger.

Milk Thistle flower essence bridges the gap between love and the lower emotions; this gap separate us from feeling love; instead we feel the lower emotions like fear, resentment, rage, anger and jealousy. For instance, Milk Thistle helps a person let go of old anger he or she may feel towards a loved one. When there is hurt inflicted by someone trusted, the feeling of betrayal can cause the emotion to run deep in the soul. Although Milk Thistle is useful for transforming many emotions that block the love vibration, it is especially indicated for those situations when one holds anger in the system. This can be conscious or unconscious anger.

Sometimes adults who were abused by a parent as children access previously unfelt anger towards the parent at a point in their lives when they are grown up and begin to understand the implications of the abuse. Milk Thistle is excellent for helping a person access these repressed feelings and to release them from the subconscious where they have done damage to the psyche in a number of ways. Milk Thistle is beneficial when one is in touch with the anger or when one knows it is appropriate to feel anger but does not feel it.

This essence helps with displaced anger, anger intensity, unconscious anger and old longstanding grudges-resentments between family members, couples or children. It is helpful in individual, couples and family therapy when there is consistent bitterness present or when anger surfaces mysteriously at the end of sessions. Although it is suggested for many individuals in counseling, it can be helpful for psychotherapists when there is difficulty with anger transference.

Energetically, the connection of the emotional or second chakra to the heart chakra is maintained. In addition, energy from the crown is brought into the heart. A person can actually transform lower emotions into loving energies with this essence. The synchronizing of these chakras also allows the release of trauma, hurt and anger. There can be cathartic releases or subtle subconscious letting go. Violent or emotional dreams can occur while taking this essence.

Milk Thistle is also useful for unexplained animosities towards certain people in our lives, who seem to inexplicably "push our buttons." These people may remind us of earlier abusive caregivers in some way or have been the actual antagonist in another lifetime. There can be nightmares associated with these individuals.

This is an essence that can be useful for adopted children who are physically abusive or who cannot control their anger. It is useful for children who are prone to violence whether or not there is a family history of violence.

Use this flower essence for any animal who has suffered abuse in the past. It is a good idea to give it as a rule to all rescued animals or even those bought in pet stores. For an animal taking Milk Thistle there is often a period of a few days where the animal is very quiet or sleeps more and stays to himself. It can also be that the animal seems to want to be around the owner more frequently. This period is usually followed by a cycle of greater energy, friendliness, playfulness and joy. Occasionally a bad tempered animal can get worse for a short period of time when taking this essence. Careful observation, extra care should be exercised. In some cases it may be necessary to restrain or confine the animal for a short period of time.

Some liver imbalances can often be an indication for the need for Milk Thistle, especially when there seems to be—in addition to the physical condition—some old anger that has not been released.

Preparation and Dosage: Add one drop of stock essence per 100 drops of neutral solution for most treatments. Add one drop of stock essence to 200 drops of neutral solution for treating animals. Use the stock essence for treating liver imbalances. It is best to prescribe this essence when a person understands how to process feelings and has built a strong support system for emotional issues.

See Also: Bull Thistle, Canada Thistle, Marshmallow, Lungwort.

MISSOURI PRIMROSE

Oenothera missouriensis

I am worthy.

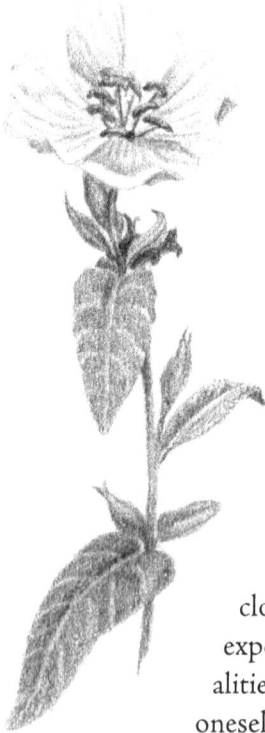

Missouri Primrose is a yellow cup-like flower that blooms in June and spreads prolifically. It grows well in either sun or shade where the brightness of the flowers display a stunning presence. The leaves, which have a red tint, are sometimes used to protect the skin from rashes or insects bites. An infusion of the blossoms has been used as an eyewash for conjunctivitis.

Indications: Has low self-esteem; is unable to receive complements; has low mineral levels; feels guilty; feels undeserving; finds fault; has eating disorder; has difficulty maintaining a primary relationship or close friendships; feels dread when things are going well; has experienced neglect or abuse; is attracted to difficult personalities and situations; has difficulty saying no or protecting oneself; resolves conflict by being "nice"; has guilt indoctrination; has learned to go without; procrastinates; sabotages self; works too much; can't see one's own talents or goodness.

Missouri Primrose works on self-esteem, helping a person learn to accept and receive love and friendship, goodness and pleasure, and other forms of self-nurturing. Self-nurturing is not exactly a natural reflex, but a conditioned response. An individual develops a sense of self-worth based on general conditions of love, respect and nurturing obtained from childhood. Receiving physical, mental, emotional and spiritual nurturing from parents, siblings, caregivers and educators conditions an individual's sense of self-worth, or the ability to *expect* a certain level of nurturing from others and from the world. This expectation is the cornerstone of an individual's self-esteem. It is through self-nurturing that a person takes in vital energies, which are later converted into confidence and drive to complete goal-directed activities.

This fundamental energetic legacy is damaged by many forms of poor child development which might include neglect, abandonment, severe punishment, abuse, guilt indoctrination, withholding love, unfairness, secrecy, strict religious upbringing or other practices which essentially rob an individual of a healthy level of self-worth and an ability to self-nurture. Many adults today are products of family, ethnic or religious training which essentially provided the basis for an under-developed sense of self-esteem.

One can test the level of this aspect of self-esteem in a number of ways: 1. The ability to make choices in one's life towards enjoyable ways of doing things like work, recreation, solitude. 2. The ability to reject activities or events that are not enjoyable. 3. The ability to choose friends and companions who are loving and nurturing. 4. The ability to accept complements when they are sincere. 5. The ability to provide a nurturing environment for one's self. Generally speaking, when one masters this aspects of living, then self-esteem and energy begin to blossom.

Adults who work too hard or too much sometimes lose touch with this fundamental truth: that self-love = self-nurturing = health = energy = wellbeing. Pushing one's self, postponing enjoyment, or even neglecting to participate in enjoyable forms of exercise or recreation can be the beginning of the erosion of the self-esteem.

Energetically, this essence helps the second chakra to take in energy. This chakra is designed to open when a person feels safe, and to draw in energy in the form of enjoyment or pleasure. When the second chakra is drawing in energy, it becomes cup-like and, in form, resembles this flower. This energy is then made available to be used by chakra three for confidence, drive, motivation, thinking, planning and activities. The more energy a person learns to take in, the more is then made available. This is how the self-esteem functions. Low self-nurturing produces little energy, which then makes it difficult to take confident, purposeful, success-driven action. Well developed self-nurturing produces a greater amount of energy, which makes success inevitable.

Relearning to perfect this energetic mechanism is the purpose of Missouri Primrose. A person taking this essence might benefit from developing an initial program of self-nurturing, making certain that there are daily pleasures being built into one's schedule, that moments of reflection, relaxation and genuine enjoyment are not bypassed because of exigency and busyness.

This essence is good for domesticated feral cats or animals who were starved by their owners. It is good for any animals that tend to eat too much. It is a good essence for oldest children, especially in family situations where the oldest child takes on adult responsibilities early. It is also good for any child who tends to take studying and preparing for the future too seriously.

Preparation and Dosage: Add one drop of the stock essence per 100 drops of neutral solution. Take this essence in a small amount of water. Use three drops per 100 drops of neutral solution when treating eating problems.

See also: Motherwort, Marshmallow, Indian Pipe.

MOTHERWORT

Leonurus cardiaca

I strengthen so that I might soften.

Motherwort is a medium sized plant common to gardens and the edges of the woodland. It is a medium sized plant with small pink flowers and very sharp seeds. Medicinally it is used for heart palpitations, hyper thyroid conditions, imbalances during menopause, for the mother after birth to stimulate the flow of milk,

Indications: Is anti-social; attracts abusive personalities; feels vulnerable; avoids most people; feels threatened; can't say no; has difficulty with certain personality types; is moody, socially fearful; has trouble in relationships; feels used by others; is seen as critical, judgmental or prejudice; feels dependent and helpless in relationships; is seen as harsh or overbearing; is cynical about relationships; is prone to endometriosis, bladder infections, sinus problems; is combative but fearful.

Motherwort flower essence teaches about and heals an aspect of the psyche that deals with hardness and softness. When we are very young our playful, carefree child-self flourishes in an atmosphere of love and protection which we traditionally receive from parents and caregivers. In such an atmosphere, inner softness remains open and accessible. When there is threat in the environment — a dysfunctional, hostile parent, for instance — the soft aspects of the psyche retreat and harden, more responsible, adult-like thinking, feeling and behaviors appear. These individuals, as adults, are often successful and very responsible, but have difficulty relaxing, having fun or being intimate, or they have hardened to the world expecting difficulty and have a personality armed to meet it.

A person needing Motherwort can also have difficulty setting boundaries in some situations, allowing themselves to be used or mistreated, especially by people they have developed some trust with. This part of the pattern keeps alive the belief that people cannot be trusted and that one should remain vigilant and mistrustful in one's life. This condition and these types of attitudes can cause or contribute to many types of health problems.

Use Motherwort in many stages of psychotherapy where the individual is learning constructive, assertive behavior to set healthy, appropriate boundaries. These outer boundaries express the being-ness of Motherwort. They provide an adult-like protection and flexibility that allow the individual to keep the inner life soft and alive. This allows for both playfulness and an awakened spiritual life.

Closing the second chakra is a reflex that happens when there is threat or even unpleasantness in the environment. This prepares the system to fire red energy upward in order to push away or separate from the difficulty. Being angry is one example of this. When there has been punishment in childhood for expressing strong feelings, this reflex is often blocked and the individual experiences difficulty in setting boundaries. Motherwort is the ideal remedy to relearn to use this reflex.

Motherwort can be helpful in treating early menopause and useful in many phases of conflict resolution, especially in couples therapy. In the later case it

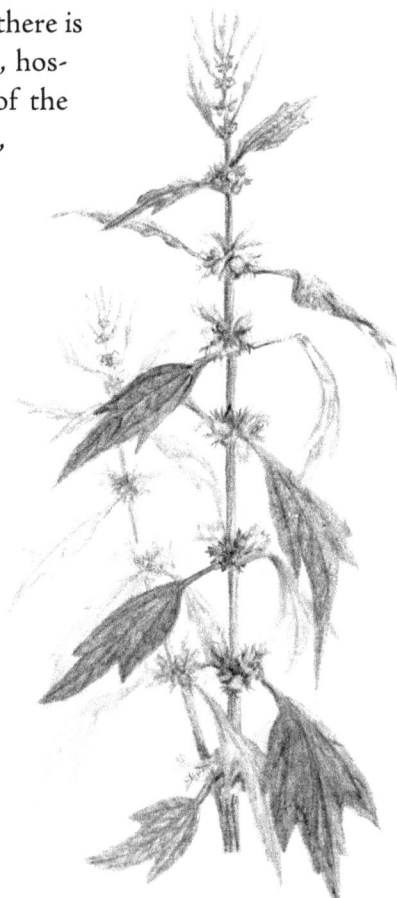

should be given to both individuals in the conflict. It is a good essence for children who have lost one or more parents and for the oldest child of each gender in any family.

Use Motherwort with animals who are very territorial or timid and fearful, with adolescents who have become moody, withdrawn or combative, with the elderly who have lost the ability to express love, and in flower essence combinations that encourage processing of difficult emotions.

Energetically, Motherwort flower essence helps the individual learn to *close* the second chakra. This is a natural reflex that children learn when they first say "no." This reflex is damaged when children are punished for expressing their independence or individuality. Upon the closing of the second chakra, the red upward channel is opened and the individual is prepared to express protective energies in the form of assertiveness, anger or action. When an individual does not have this ability, there is a general sense of vulnerability and unease, especially around people.

Preparation and Dosage: Add one drop of stock essence per 100 drops of neutral solution for most treatments. Add one drop of stock essence per 200 drops of neutral solution for treating animals.

See Also: Marshmallow, Milk Thistle, Lungwort.

*   *   *

> *Wondrous truths and manifold as wondrous,*
> *God hath written in the stars above,*
> *But not less in the bright flowers under us*
> *Stands the revelation of His love.*
>
> — Longfellow

ONION

Allium cepa

I release sadness and embrace joy.

Onion is an edible bulb that produces white flowers in the late spring. It is used for flavoring in cooking and as an expectorating herb for lung infections such as colds, bronchitis, fevers. It is popularly used as a cough syrup and externally as a lung poultice. It is also used for digestive problems, water retention, and circulation problems.

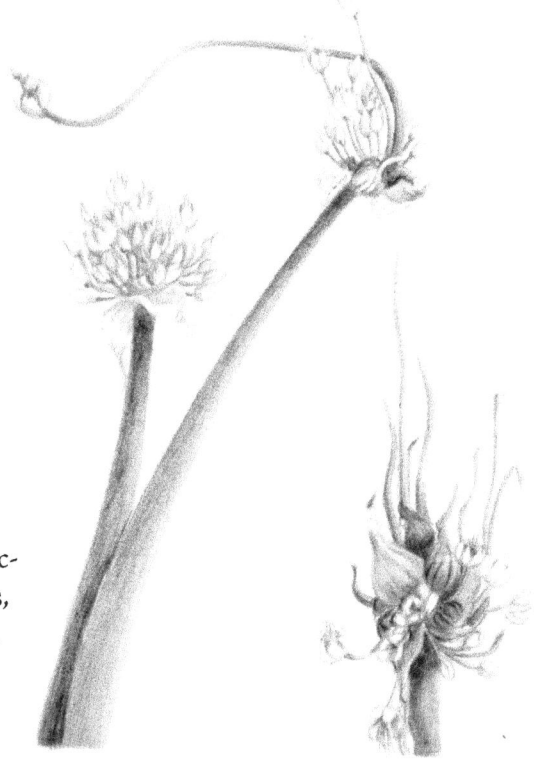

Indications: Has unresolved grief, unexpressed sadness; is reluctant or unable to cry; is weepy; can't concentrate; can't focus; has low energy; has mucous or water retention; has difficulty breathing; has puscular psoriasis; has edema; is susceptible to colds; is bitter; cynical, angry or frustrated; cries all the time.

Onion flower essence assists in all aspects of the grieving process, helping a person, first to access the emotion which is present, then to express it deeply and completely, and then to move the grief-emotion present out of the system. In initial stages of grief, this may be anger or frustration. Or it may be an intense wave of sadness. Onion helps move the grieving process quickly and gently from the initial to the final stages.

We are now discovering how important it is for mental, physical and emotional health for feelings to be fully accessed and expressed. This importance was not always recognized. With earlier generations, and in some cultures more than others, expressing of emotions was seen as a sign of weakness, preference being given to showing those states of being which were considered socially appropriate. Onion is advisable for those who are relearning about the value of expressing feelings.

Onion is appropriate to take either as a companion to a present situation evoking grieving, such as the death of a loved one, or to release past grief which one has suppressed. At times, the release of old feelings can be an intense experience. For this reason, it is good to enlist coaching or support from friends and professionals while taking Onion. This can be especially true for men who have been conditioned to not show the emotion of sadness.

Onion can accelerate the psychotherapeutic process, helping an individual move more quickly through the various stages and levels of awareness and release. It is also an excellent support for children who tend to be very emotional. Onion, in this case, provides a strengthening, allowing emotions to complete their natural cycle. Here it should be given once daily or every other day. Over time a stabilizing of emotions or an increased maturity will be observed.

Treatment of somatic symptoms from early suppressed grief can be complemented with Onion flower essence. These include stomach and heart problems, as well as certain types of skin imbalances where there is a weeping rash or sores such as with puscular psoriasis.

The signature of the plant is both in its relation to the wateriness of the bulb and of the stinging heat which affects the eyes. Onion flower essence harmonizes the relationship of the fire chakra (chakra three) and the water chakra (chakra two). When there is grief or sadness, chakras two and three work together much like a forced-water heating system. Chakra three heats up and begins drawing the watery emotions upward. Weeping is one way this process expresses in the body. It is nature's way of cleansing, purifying the system.

Onion is a good flower essence to use with animals who have been mistreated, especially those that tend to whine for no apparent reason. It is wise to use this essence for animals who have lost a mate, an animal friend or human companion. It is also good to use when the animal's caretaker is grieving the loss of a friend or family member.

For young children, this essence prevents unconscious fears of death and loss from lodging in the personality. With older children and adolescents, it can prevent or treat the acting out of anger that can follow loss or the death of someone close.

Preparation and Dosage: Add one drop of stock essence per 100 drops of neutral solution for most treatments. Add one drop of stock essence per 200 drops of neutral solution for treating animals. It is best to take this essence in a small amount of water.

See Also: Milk Thistle, Lungwort.

PINK AMARANTHUS

Amaranthus hypochondriacus

I trust in the power of love.

The pink variety of this plant has somewhat larger and thicker flowers than the golden variety. These bloom in the summer and offer a stunning spectacle in any garden. The drooping flower speaks about surrender, gaining strength and power in yielding. The pink represents the softness of the heart.

Indications: Experiences patterns of failure in relationships; is love addicted, obsessive or aggressive in pursuit of relationships; fears being hurt; has overly-high standards for relationship; feels anxiety or dread in relation to love; chooses "safe" partners; is antagonistic or plaintive with partners; hits or slaps others; has low tolerance for mistakes or shortcomings of friends or partners; allows abuse by others to continue.

The challenge of relationships today has made many people reluctant to enter committed partnerships. Those who have felt abused, jaded, betrayed in relationships, can develop attitudes and reflexes, which can prevent relationships from developing. Although these reflexes are essentially protective in nature, they can also serve to confuse a person as to what is really going on as s/he fails again and again at attempts to form healthy partnerships.

Like Golden Amaranthus this flower essence fosters a feeling of safety, its specialty being safety within the heartspace. This essence gives us a lesson in the power of love. It is for people afraid to open the heart for fear of vulnerability, weakness, hurt. Learning to trust love as an active force in one's life strengthens, nurtures and heals.

Those needing Pink Amaranthus will show either the tendency to avoid partnership altogether or to be overly willful in the pursuit of a relationship. In the second case, it is often part of the pattern to pursue a new relationship too

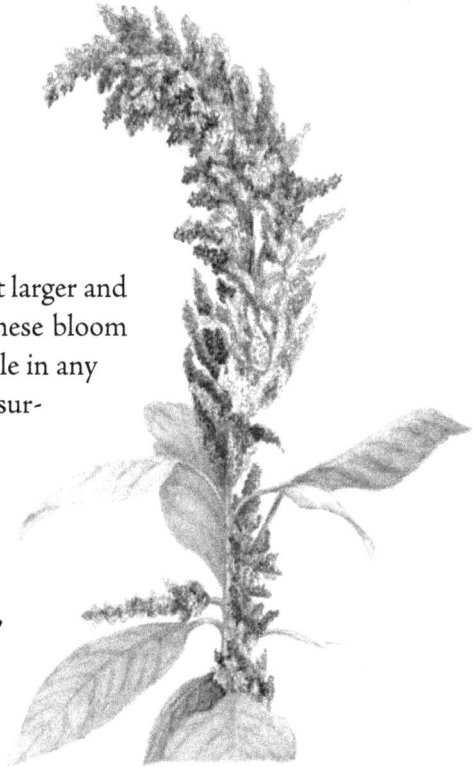

soon after ending a previous one. Unconscious feelings of insecurity, guilt or failure from the previous relationship are often stronger than the instinct to wait until the healing and lessons are processed. These feelings of guilt and failure create a tendency to "try again" rather than be reflective and heal some of the deeper issues of the past relationship. In this situation new relationships can begin and end quickly, deepening the frustrations until a polarization (between wanting to be in a healthy relationship and not believing it will ever happen) causes a person to begin to confuse feelings of love with many other negative emotions which surface simultaneously with an attraction to another.

Pink Amaranthus helps with many problems surrounding the search for partnership, first by bringing fears and negative experiences to the conscious level where they can be worked on, and then by providing energies which can assist in creating healthy feelings and attitudes surrounding relationship. Thus, a person seeking partnership is aware of and utilizes the positive love energies that are available rather than focusing on fears, doubts and negativity.

This essence energetically allows the second chakra, the relationship chakras to receive energies from the upper chakras. The heart, which is located between these two polarities, becomes more a part of the energetic rhythm. This allows a person to feel less troubled about relationships in general, and to make wiser choices in specific relationships. A general shift in attitudes about relationship comes about through a cleansing of the second chakra which happens naturally as higher energies come in. This cleansing is best undertaken with supportive psychotherapy. It is also recommended that new relationships be avoided temporarily while this essence is being used. This is because the initial action of the essence may bring up parental imprints around relationship at the same time that the heart is being stimulated. In some cases this can cause confusion, the new relationship acting as an anchor point or metaphor for these old energies.

Consider this essence for: teenagers who have poor attitudes about relationships, especially those who have parents who do not have a healthy partnership, adults who are considering entering relationship after a period of being alone, animals who have been abused or abandoned and are relearning to trust a new owner, especially dogs who have very affectionate natures and children who have difficulty making friends.

Preparation and Dosage: One drop of stock essence per 100 drops of neutral solution. Take a few drops of this 2-3 times per day.

See Also: Wood Betony, Blackberry Lily, Star Jasmine.

PINK LADY'S SLIPPER

Cypripedium acaule

The power of the Light lives
within me

A stunning wild ground orchid, this plant, because of its beauty, rarity, and resistance to cultivation, has reached the endangered list in many states. Although it grows prolifically in forest areas where conditions are perfect, it literally disappears in civilized areas. The flower essence of this plant was made without picking the flowers.

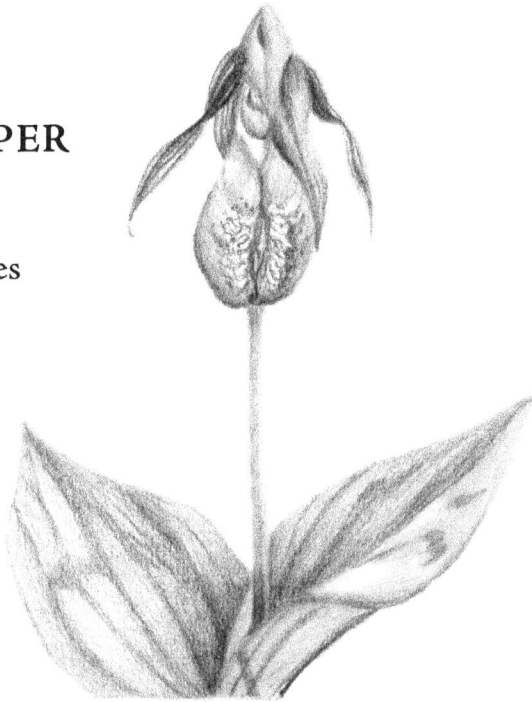

Indications: Feels alienated; feels social frustrations; is over-sensitive; has headaches; has sore feet or ankles; has digestive problems; feels uncertain about goals; feels depressed; is rebellious; has suicidal thoughts; has obsessive thoughts; is fatigued; has low motivation; has identity crisis or mid-life crisis; has low self-esteem; is a late starter; has bursts of energy; has flashes of genius; doesn't fit in; hears a different drummer; dislikes school.

Pink Lady's Slipper flower essence carries the paradox of the plant, for although this flower is one of exquisite delicateness and rare beauty, it is also one that contains a powerful vibration. It is as if the plant is able to act as a focal point for the mysterious power of the forest.

The very appearance of Lady's Slipper is, in itself, a paradox. It appears to some as very feminine because of its delicate presentation. Others see maleness, even sexuality in the plant. Some see the lightness or air nature while others see the opposite and its relationship to the earth and to the feet. All of these are quite correct and part of the signature of bringing the masculine and feminine aspects of power together and also of the ethereal qualities alive in the personality which need grounding, understanding and expression.

In the world today, power and force are almost synonymous. Those people or groups that are able to exert the most outward force are considered the most powerful. Gentleness and subtlety, although somewhat appreciated, are identified more with weakness than power. Yet looking closer, we can see many examples of the powerful influence of art, beauty, and forms of power that are by no means overt. There are many examples in myths and in history of wars fought over beauty or major political decisions and moves guided by subtle intelligence rather than by bravado. Pink Lady's Slipper is an essence that supports and strengthens those individuals who embody this special kind of subtle or less overt power. This can include artistic types, mathematical or technological genius, and altruistic or spiritually minded people. All of these types possess a certain type of real, practical, but subtle power.

Those people who feel a knowledge or wisdom within them or a deep love or joy, but feel reluctant to express this part of them will benefit from Lady's Slipper. It is as if the power of the plant begins to vibrate within them, adding strength to that deep feeling of being special—making it more available to the conscious mind for expression.

The powers of subtlety, wisdom, genius, art, love, and joy are not merely philosophical or conceptual. They are real and present powers living deeper in the psyche, needing a certain type of circumstance or environment in order to thrive and develop. This is another flower essence that connects upper to lower chakras. Here the third or identity chakra is given added information from the crown and brow chakras. Information from the upper chakras is usually held "in reserve" until the development of the lower chakras signals a readiness to receive the information. With Pink Lady's Slipper, more of this information makes its way down for awareness and use.

Many children today are not fitting into the framework of our educational system which—although history has taught us otherwise—glorifies a more overt, even physical type of power but gives less value to the subtle, the academic, the artistic. Our systems are no longer serving the masses of the new generation with present attitudes and educational values. Indeed, many suffer from a feeling of alienation within the structures of public and private education. Higher sensitivities are not stimulated, challenged or in many cases even recognized. It is as if the system does not know how to satisfy the longing in the souls of these young individuals. Consider this flower essence a complementary treatment for any therapy or alternative educational activity exploring deeper meanings and values with young people.

Adults who feel out of step with their partners, friends, and associates, and who have always felt somehow that their lives were meant to be the expression of something deeper would benefit from this essence, as would those who are finding their "real" careers later in life. This applies to many new-age health practitioners today who go through periods of self-doubt about their direction and value. Pink lady's Slipper can do wonders to relieve some of these symptoms and to strengthen the light within them.

Many physical, mental, and emotional conditions associated with these circumstances can be treated with Pink Lady's Slipper: depression, energy loss, boredom, recurring headaches, sleeplessness, nervousness, frustration, alienation, rebelliousness, inflammations, as well as weaknesses in the legs, hips, and lower organs. It is important to understand that the essence represents not so much a cure for these symptoms but rather a longer-term evolutionary therapy, which can ease many of the problems that the deep thinking, the brilliant, the artistic and the spiritually minded face in society today.

All household, caged or shelter animals will feel the benefits of this essence. It is a tonic, which can improve both temperament and physical functioning.

Preparation and Dosage: One drop of the stock essence per 100 in a dosage bottle for animals; two drops per 100 for children; three drops per 100 for adults. When treating physical symptoms in animals add two more drops per 100. For physical symptoms in people, use the stock frequency. Administer three drops under the tongue 2-3 times per day.

See Also: White Columbine, Lovage.

*   *   *

There are philosophies as varied as the flowers of the field,
and some of them weeds and a few of them poisonous weeds.
But they none of them create the psychological conditions
in which I first saw, or desired to see, the flower.

— G. K. Chesterton

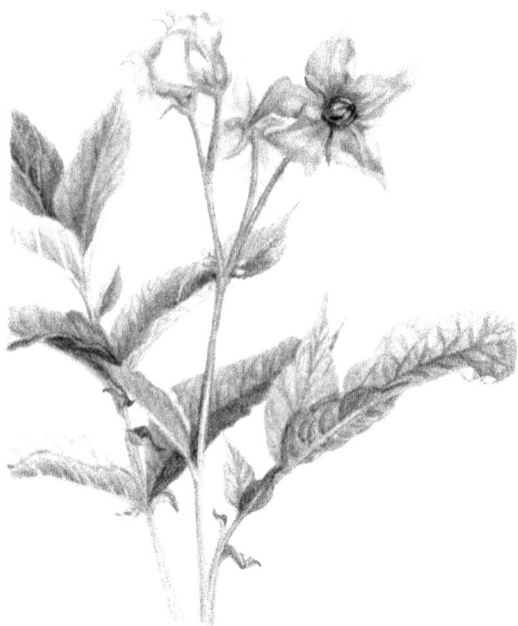

POTATO

Solanum tuberosum

I am here. I am now.

Potato is part of the night-shade family. The flowers are white and yellow and open in four directions. The tuber is a popular food staple and it is used herbally as a poultice and to soothe hemorrhoids. Sometimes potato is prescribed to remove cysts.

Indications: Is spacey, un-grounded, fanciful; has daydreams; can't manifest; is attracted to highs; is not practical; is unable to see whole picture; talks excessively; is abstract; is cold in extremities; is delusional; avoids difficult emotions; has addictive personality; can't cope.

Often spirituality is confused with blissful or expansive states, rather than practical and experiential wisdom. An individual, for instance, may be seeking a spiritual life, being attracted exclusively to those people, places and things that produce a "high." Real spirituality attempts to ground and integrate spiritual impulses or truths into the whole psyche. Rather than being always euphoric, there are many stages of internal and external work necessary to make spirituality real.

Potato flower essence expresses the balance of grounding and expanding, of being in the body and in expansive states. It helps a person "bring in" or make real, new experiences. For this reason it is useful to use Potato flower essence after any deep healing or expansive experience. It gently brings the person back into the body, into their "normal reality" where they can reflect about the experience, integrate it and then act.

This essence also helps people who are very intellectual or spiritually inclined and less "in touch" with more mundane matters. There can be inability to cope with stress or to experience emotions. There can also be a generally fearful or timid nature. Here the action of Potato brings one more into the present, into the body where one is more in touch with one's physical and emotional issues.

This is a good essence for stabilizing one's spiritual development so that it continues at an uninterrupted pace. It provides a foundation for balanced mental and spiritual growth, and can be useful for many who have genuine spiritual experiences or flashes of genius.

It is helpful for children who are very imaginative and sometimes become confused about what is real or prefer to stay in their imaginations for undue periods of time. It is also useful for gifted children who develop a talent or a strong intellect at a rapid pace. Here it helps children keep a foundation and perspective that is healthy, so that their development can proceed.

Potato flower essence stabilizes the base chakra. Higher thoughts, inspired ideas, creative impulses are all connected to and influenced by the practical side of a person. What one conceives of automatically references what is real in this realm. This prevents dreamy, escapist fantasies or delusional thinking.

Use Potato when reintroducing a wild animal back into nature. This includes animals who were taken in and cared for because of an injury, or animals who were born in captivity and are being released. Although the process may take slightly longer with Potato, it is likely to be less stressful for the animal thereby increasing the chances for successful rehabilitation.

Preparation and Dosage: One drop of the stock essence per hundred in a dosage bottle for most treatments. Take a few drops of this 2-3 times a day.

See Also: Habanero Pepper, Onion, Lemon Balm.

*   *   *

God grows weary of great kingdoms, but never of little flowers.

— anon

SCARLET PIMPERNEL

Anagalis arvensis

My past lives in my present.

A low-growing, spreading annual.
The tiny flowers are usually scarlet
with a purple center. It has been called
"poor man's weatherglass" because the flowers are very
sensitive, opening to the sun and remaining closed on
rainy and cloudy days. A tincture of the plant is used to
treat skin eruptions and ulcers. It is also used as a diuretic.

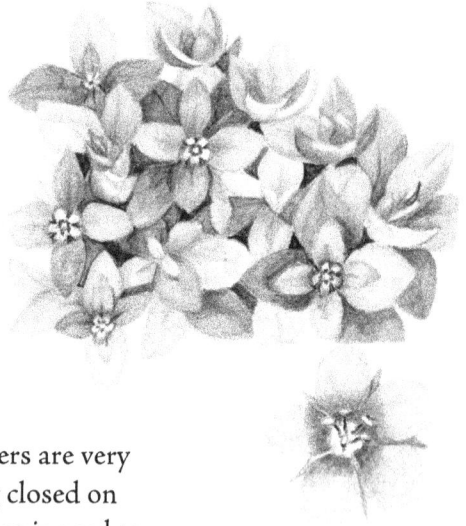

Indications: Is tense or anxious; avoids talking about the past; tends to be controlled; has trouble with addictive behavior; avoids feeling intense emotions; is susceptible to inflammations; can be lethargic; has strong attitudes; acts out on occasion; can have anger attacks; has scalp or skin rashes.

Hurt, anger, sadness, grief, resentment, trauma from the past, all have a way of finding a hiding place in the psyche and a way of co-existing with more conscious values and attitudes. There is a kind of balance and agreement that happens between the conscious and the unconscious, resulting in a personality adaptation that favors the present and avoids the past. Subconscious debris stays hidden for the most part, and uses the attitudes to make a place for them. For instance, there can be a belief that it is perfectly right to dislike, even hate certain people or types. The attitude is, in part, the puppet of deeper, more hidden, trauma-type imprints. The deeper imprints become the fuel for the beliefs or attitudes. The dislike or hatred comes from an imprint of the past which is still active but buried in the psyche; the beliefs are convenient justifications for allowing the feelings to express themselves.

At any given moment, a person strives to balance the deeper feelings with what his or her beliefs are. In some cases, beliefs are formed to justify feelings, in other cases a person works to change feelings that do not fit with beliefs. This striving-for-balance in the system can be deadly when the belief system is constructed to allow toxic, subconscious realities to live in the system. Here the person indulges in delusions that there is a good reason to have negative feelings, hurtful intentions or evil deeds. Many disturbances in the personality can be described in this way.

Scarlet Pimpernel is a powerful catalyst, and for this reason it should be used with caution. At any given time, it can help a person develop a healthier balance between attitudes and feelings. It does this by first, stimulating more hidden layers of the emotional body. A person has easier access to deeper feelings. With some work, a person can move these toxic vibrations out of the system, which in turn, makes it more possible to develop attitudes and behaviors which are healthier. This process takes time and must be done in stages. It also usually requires some complementary psychotherapy and release work. It is, as one can imagine, an excellent remedy which can be used for those who are in prison rehabilitation programs and for teens whose acting out becomes self-destructive.

Scarlet Pimpernel flower essence is helpful for those who have done some inner work but are somewhat frustrated by a lull in the process. It is as if there is something there to work on but it is not entirely within reach. Taking this essence helps a person re-engage with core emotional issues which then can be addressed and released.

Energetically, Scarlet Pimpernel stimulates the deeper layers of the lower chakras. These layers can be near motionless most of the time, as they contain dormant energies of the past that are generally suppressed. Slight movement of these layers can stimulate these energies to become active and to begin circulating into the conscious system. The circulation of these energies into the conscious system can cause a variety of responses depending on how ready the person is to receive the new-old information. The red channel between the chakras is stimulated; violent or emotional dreams, drama, and slight, temporary inflammations are some possible initial responses to this essence. On the other hand this essence can ease any of these symptoms if they are already present.

This is a good essence to use for children who are withdrawn or who tend towards sulking. It can, with some professional guidance, promote better communication with them. Use this essence with animals who have lost a companion pet or who are sullen, lethargic or depressed, or with rescued animals who have a susceptibility to rashes or inflammations.

Preparation and Dosage: One drop of the stock per 100 drops in a dosage bottle for most treatments. Use up to 10 drops per 100 if there are inflammations present during the treatment period.

See Also: Fraxinella, Milk Thistle, Onion, Bull Thistle.

SKULLCAP

Scuttellaria laterifolia

I am with others like myself.

Skullcap is a low-growing perennial herb with blue or violet flowers. It is used herbally to treat nerve disorders.

Indications: Feels alone; can't relate; can't socialize; feels prejudice; is antisocial, judgmental, out of touch with self; feels self-hatred; displays self-neglect; avoids others; is aloof; is at odds with friends; can't accept self; has tics; feels social anxiety; needs to be alone.

This essence teaches a valuable if not metaphysical lesson about socialization. In its first action, the essence teaches one to be in touch with one's self. For this alone it is a valuable essence for recovery when one's essential self has retreated from consciousness. Here it provides a kind of bridge back to the treasure chest of one's truer nature. One's feelings, interests, preferences and self-nurturing abilities are regained.

In its second action, Scullcap sensitizes one to others. From a place of certainty about one's own self, there is then a greater ability to extend sensitivity, understanding, and compassion to others. The lesson here is clear: true understanding and compassion come from a place of self-understanding and self-nurturing.

The speed and stress of daily living, the bombardment of the mind with stimulation, early pain and trauma — can all conspire against the natural sensitivity of the soul. Within this context, it is almost inevitable that the psyche retreats and grows insensitive to many important issues in life. The natural caring, joy, sadness, indignation or outrage that can be felt keenly in the soul from observing daily life events and situations are often replaced by a retreat and resignation or a numbness and shock.

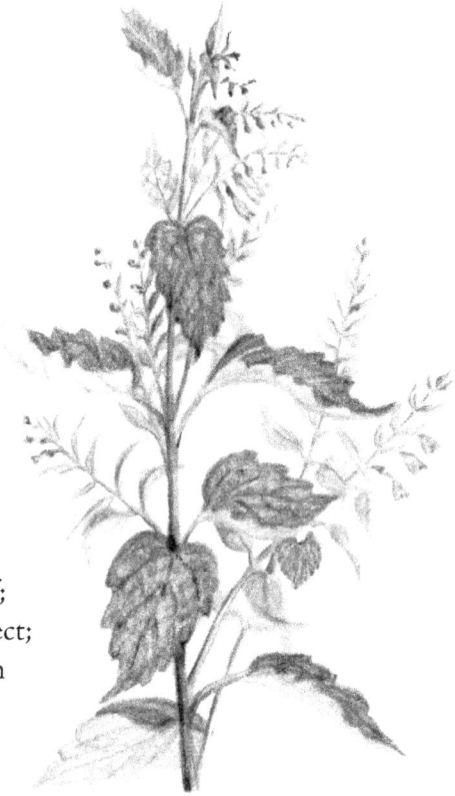

Skullcap allows the soul's natural sensitivities to the self and to others to open, both for specific short-term purposes, and as part of a longer-term therapeutic process of healing damaged self-esteem. With Skullcap one learns about feeling one's state of being in each moment. This gives one the ability to improve self-esteem through improved moment-to-moment self-care.

Professionals who heal others could benefit from Skullcap. It sharpens sensitivities to others thereby promoting a stronger bond and consequently, healing potential. It is especially beneficial to use with those clients who are more difficult for the professional to connect with. In this case the feeling of connection helps lessen judgment or other feelings, which promote separation and prevent effectiveness.

Energetically, Scullcap stimulates the blue, or downward channel, which connects all the chakras. This manner of mild stimulation provides a temporary integration to chakras one two and three, which then telegraph messages of safety and connection throughout the nervous system. This solidity in the system is further emphasized in the strengthening of the entire field, which is held tight by the harmony of the lower chakras. The result is a feeling of increased safety, sense of self and consequently increased ability to connect with others.

Skullcap is helpful for teenagers who often become self-absorbed, cynical and very selective and guarded about friendships. During this period there may be an increased insensitivity to others in the household or a general self-neglect around matters of health and safety. Small children who are very inward and strike out unexpectedly at others could benefit from Skullcap. It is an excellent complement to PTS therapy when one has retreated inwardly following a shock or trauma. Use it as an essence to help with rehabilitation in prison reform. Use it also as an aid to recovery for women who have given up children for adoption or who have had abortions.

Skullcap is helpful for traumatized animals that are overly aggressive; it is helpful for animals who are gentle with their caregivers but prone to attacking others. In both these cases it is important to use the essence in conjunction with training, behavior modification, and other animal behavior therapies.

Preparation and Dosage: One drop of the stock essence per hundred in a dosage bottle for animals. Two drops per hundred for children. Three drops per hundred for adults.

See Also: Golden Amaranthus, Hemp Agrimony, Motherwort.

SOLOMON'S SEAL

Polygonatum odoratum

I accept.

This is a particularly lovely plant which
bends earthward with bell-like green
and white blooms. The leaves are a
rich green and the roots have chain-
like links reminding one of the spine. This
plant grows in the woods but a larger more
showy version has been cultivated for gardens.
Herbally, the root tincture is used to treat a wide
variety of problems relating to tendons, ligaments,
joints, bruises, breaks and calcifications.

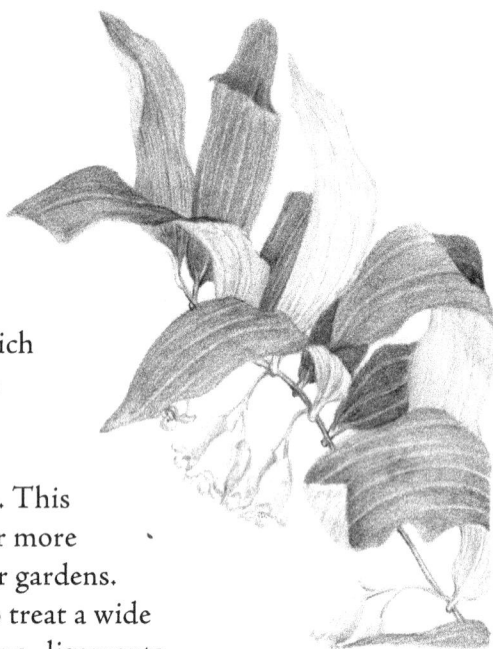

Indications: Is easily frustrated; is bothered by imperfection; gives up easily;
avoids competition; is not a good loser; rejects structure and authority but
longs for true leadership; is drawn to escapism and addictions; avoids planning; is regularly disappointed; has problems with knee, joints or lower back;
is moody.

When things go wrong or do not work out, the personality learns many
ways of reacting, coping, responding, adapting. In fact it is within this day-to-
day testing that the soul learns about issues that form the foundation of a
healthy personality and a happy life. Solomon's Seal helps the individual learn
to let go of the control or attachment to outcomes, learning to refocus and
adapt to mishaps rather than react with anger and frustration. Of course there
is always a human and understandable level of attachment to outcomes, which
will result in natural feelings of disappointment and frustration when things
do not work out the way we want. However, when we know that there is nothing that can be done to change what has already happened, the most healthy
alternative is to reconsider the situation, reform plans, reset goals, change
expectations.

This may not be as easy as it sounds. There is a kind of grieving that each
person must engage in before this process of resetting goals can be complete,

letting go of the attachment to the previously held reality or expectation, and seeing the benefit of changing one's orientation. This type of process can happen in a few moments. A person feels frustration and lets go of it, seeing a more beneficial possibility in continuing in an adapted manner.

Business leaders today know the value of this skill to refocus and adapt to situations that do not work out. The most successful companies are those that have learned to roll with the punches, learn from mistakes and to constantly adapt to fluctuations, surprises and changes that can not be foreseen or controlled. On the personal level, the lesson is the same. Survival and happiness require an understanding of how to respond regularly to the changing variables of life.

Solomon's Seal is a treatment for personalities that have difficulty letting go of attachment to results or outcomes, reacting with anger and frustration rather than with understanding, skill and flexibility. It can also be helpful for those who lower their standards to prevent the pain of disappointment or to protect themselves from their own volatility. It is useful in times when one does not know whether to let go or push on when things are beginning to indicate an unwanted outcome is probable.

Energetically, flexibility comes from a healthy second chakra and emotional body. A person who allows the full range of emotions will more easily reach a level of acceptance when frustration arises. Acceptance is the ability of the second chakra to receive higher impulses from upper chakras or "rise above" the emotions of the lower nature. Solomon's Seal helps the second chakra stay in touch with the higher impulses of the upper chakras and in this way steers the individual away from frustration and towards accepting lessons available.

There is a strengthening that comes from the flexibility that this essence produces. It is as if one becomes more poised and ready to deal with any outcome rather than depend on a single one. The context becomes broader, problem solving takes on another level, a person can become alive and excited over things not working out because of the energy that is brought to the surface.

This remedy can be helpful for finicky cats, or for any animal who resists learning new behaviors.

Preparation and Dosage: One drop of stock essence per 100 in a dosage bottle.

See Also: Golden Amaranthus, Blue Vervain.

STAR JASMINE

Trachelosperumum
jasminoides

I am lifted.

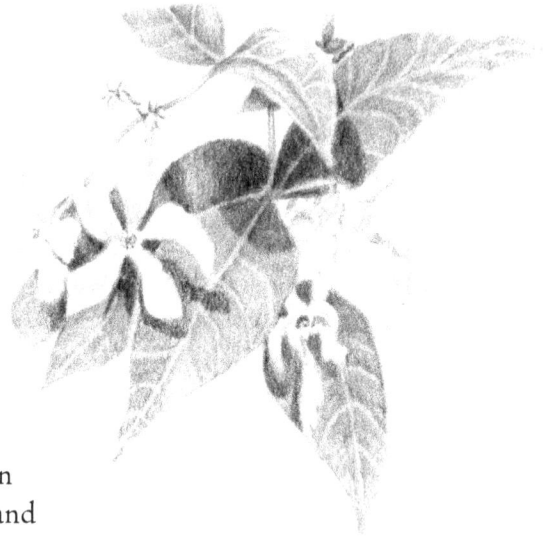

Star Jasmine is a tropical vine
that produces fragrant flowers in
the spring and summer. It produces an
aromatic oil which is used in tantra and
for uplifting the downcast spirits.

Indications: Feels hopeless, agnostic, fatalistic, cynical, depressed, overwhelmed, materialistic, narrow minded, uninspired, blocked, sad, lonely; feels
heavy; cannot think clearly; is congested frequently.

Star Jasmine flower essence has an uplifting quality which is useful in many
circumstances. It is useful for those who are doing emotional work and enter a
period of low energy or heaviness. It is universally applicable for somberness,
fatigue from working a daily routine, low-level depression or stress from a regular and constant frustration. It can help those who feel morose, hopeless,
dejected, fatalistic, cynical or negative.

Star Jasmine has universal applications for enhancing the intellect and spir-
itualizing the thinking process. This means added clarity to strictly intellectual
pursuits and increased insight and illumination to areas where the intellect
receives inspiration from the intuition. Here the thinking process becomes less
bound by rules, precedent or attitudes. This is a good essence to prescribe for
artists, inventors or managers who are looking for more inspiration in their
problem solving processes.

Because of its generally upward nature, Star Jasmine combines well with
many other essences that stimulate the processing of lower suppressed
emotions. Essences that allow processing can induce short periods of
withdrawal and heaviness. Jasmine supports and lightens processing so that
there can be an understanding as old feelings are reckoned with and released.

Star Jasmine reconnects the upper chakras to the lower ones. This
increases the ability of the higher centers to uplift the lower three. The higher

frequencies of chakra six and seven are strengthened as they pull energy upwards from the lower centers in their quest to spiritualize them. This is how Star Jasmine is able to uplift or add a spiritual perspective to many functions. Sexuality, for instance, becomes more integrated with higher ideals, emotions become more aligned with spirituality, love becomes more unconditional.

This is a useful essence for healers of all kinds, especially for psychotherapists and those who work directly with observable dysfunction who may occasionally feel depressed, overwhelmed or even fatalistic from having such close and regular association with these energies. Jasmine helps keep one's point of view from being lowered.

Star Jasmine helps very serious, responsible or mature children maintain their childlike, joyful nature. It is also useful for all pets who experience a lethargy or depression, especially larger animals, as these tend to feel their own weight as part of a lower mood. This includes large dogs, horses and many wild animals in captivity.

Preparation and Dosage: One drop of the stock essence per 100 in a dosage bottle for most cases.

See Also: Borage.

STINGING NETTLE

Urtica dioica

I release the pain of the past.

This is a popular herb with drooping, pendulous flowers. The tiny hairs on the leaves and stem produce a sting when they are touched. It is used as a highly nutritional and mineral-rich tonic and as a medicinal herb to treat kidney-related illnesses, prostate enlargement, adrenal gland problems, and allergies. The stimulating stings are used to renew nerve function and relieve arthritis.

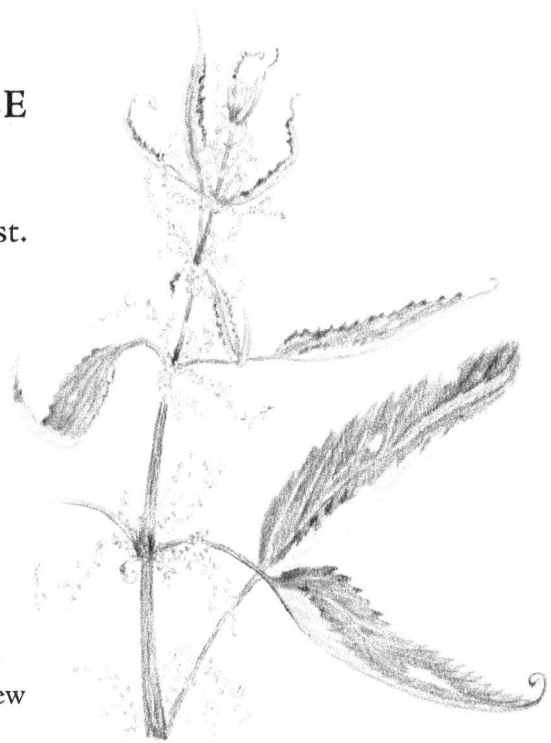

Indications: Has a tendency towards drama; is very emotional; expresses rage, torment, confusion or grief; is fearful when things are going well; believes that life is not fair; is cynical about people; is a crusader for just causes; holds suppressed rage; lashes out unexpectedly; is addicted to drugs or alcohol; is a workaholic; has difficulty forming healthy relationships; pushes people away; has low or damaged self-esteem; is abusive to others; has social fears; wants to get into a relationship when alone, and then wants to be alone when in a relationship.

Stinging Nettle helps ease pain in the present that is intensified or skewed from untreated early childhood pain. Psychotherapists call this "carried feeling reality" since what is felt in the present is really something from the past that has been triggered into surfacing. An individual may feel rage instead of anger or intense grief instead of sadness. Or a person may feel an emotional state without there being any obvious trigger in the present. It can be as if the person is overcome by some emotion for no reason at all. For these individuals, there is generally a sense of being misunderstood, shunned or judged by others since the state is so subjective, and others cannot relate to the intensity of or the reason for the reactions they are witnessing.

Stinging Nettle has many applications to the psychotherapeutic process that is anchored in the relationship of the past to the present. Here the use of the flower essence can greatly accelerate associations made between early childhood pain and present stresses and difficulties. Stinging Nettle can also be ideal for family therapy when those who were traumatized as children have reached adulthood and begin to re-explore early family dysfunction in a couples or family therapy setting. In this case it is these adults in the family who can benefit most from taking Stinging Nettle.

Stinging Nettle is also an elixir to ease any type of emotional pain experienced in the present. This includes pain from being offended, picked on, misunderstood, or pain from more intense situations such as physical abuse or torment. It is a good essence to use with adopted children, children from broken homes and children whose parents are going through separation and divorce.

Energetically the action of Stinging Nettle is deep. The downward growing flowers and the sharp pain from the sting indicate its influence on deeper repressed areas of the psyche contained in chakras one, two and three. These areas tend to be responsible for irrational responses to people or situations that "trigger" the individual. These areas in the lower layers of the chakras are awakened by this essence. In this way a person can become more aware of the basis of his or her irrational responses and begin working with the deeper personal issues rather that degenerating to externalizing and blaming.

This is another essence to use with animals from shelters or those who have been punished or beaten. It helps animals better discriminate between situations of safety and those of threat. An added ease and calmness will often be observed. In many cases, dogs who begin taking this essence may sleep more or become less social for a short period of time. After this an increased strength and socialness may be noticeable.

Preparation and Dosage: One drop of the stock essence per hundred in a dosage bottle for animals or children. Two drops per 100 for adults.

See Also: Milk Thistle, Bull Thistle, Canada Thistle, Scarlet Pimpernel.

SUMAC

Rhus glabra

My faith carries me.

Sumac is a shrub or small tree that bears green flowers which turn to red in the fall and remain on the plant throughout the winter. It is used herbally to stimulate the rhythmic system and to strengthen the blood.

Indications: Wants to quit; is resigned; has loss of faith; feels hopeless; feels like giving up; has lost motivation; has no stamina; is losing heart; feels discouragement; thinks life is meaningless; is anemic; feels that life has passed by.

Those projects or enterprises we invest most of our time, resources and energy in are usually those that have deeper meaning to us. As values change for an individual over the course of time or as obstacles arise, there are bound to be times when the operating principles behind our lives are challenged, even shaken.

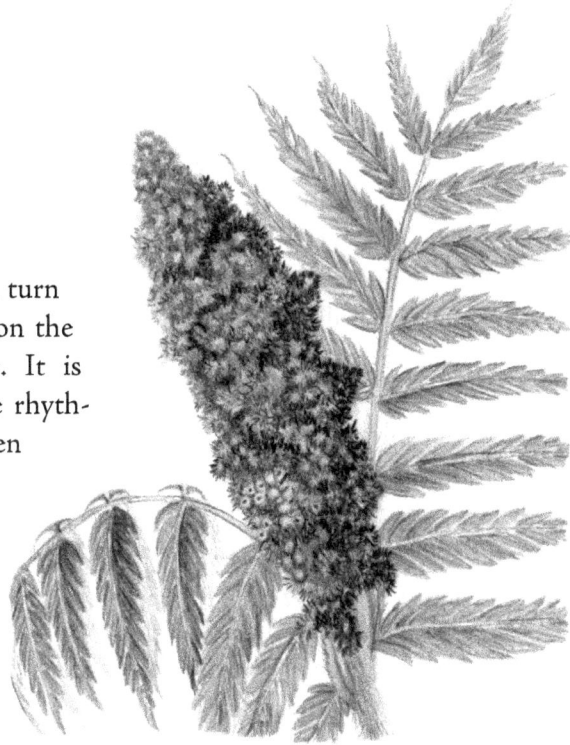

Sumac teaches the lesson of striving and endurance. It helps the soul feel the value of what is held in the heart as important and to use it as energy. The meaning of time and duration begin to mean less when the perspective of value comes from something real in the heart. Accessing this energy is what keeps us working through difficult times.

Sumac is helpful for those times when we feel like giving up. This can relate to a short-term project, to life goals or to an internal attitude. For instance, a person may feel that all his or her efforts to succeed in a career have been in vain — that it is time to give up the fight. Or a person may feel discouraged about spiritual goals that no longer seem attainable. This is different from making a decision to regroup, rethink or re-strategize. A person needing Sumac feels he or she has lost the heart and soul of the struggle; the meaning for continuing seems to have gone.

Sumac is helpful to use when one is deciding about a long-term life investment such as a college education or a "back to school" project later in life. It helps those who have difficulty feeling the energy to look and plan so far ahead.

In early years, children may begin to find deeper values that provide motivation for projects and then become discouraged when they do not feel their efforts have had an impact. In this case, Sumac helps the child "feel" the value of the work even when the physical or social impact might not be readily observable. This is an essence to use for mid-life crises or for any time that discouragement or disillusionment causes a person to go inward to re-evaluate. It is an excellent essence to take at the onset of retirement or any time there is a major life change.

Energetically, Sumac strengthens the base chakra and its ability to hold a foundational rhythm for the other chakras. It is slightly uplifted when it connects to the heart chakra. This rhythm is used by the whole system to sustain drive and energy. It is this rhythm that the individual learns to rely on to continue striving or working towards any goal.

This essence can be used as a general tonic for animals entering old age. It is especially useful for animals who become "retired," or no longer able to keep up some of their previous routines with their caregivers.

Preparation and Dosage: Three drops of stock essence per 100 of neutral solution for most cases. Take a few drops of this 2-3 times a day.

See Also: Borage, Lovage.

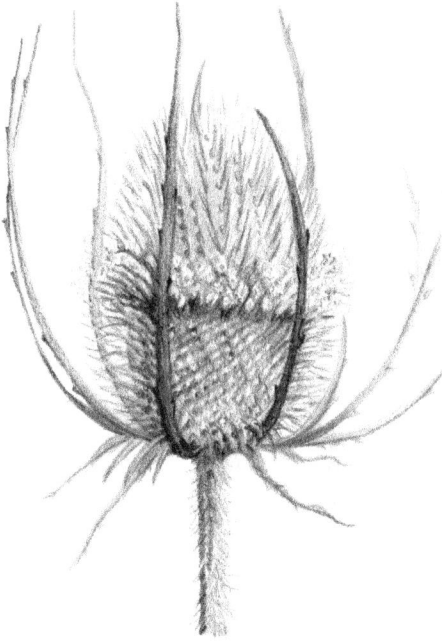

TEASEL

Dipsacus sativus

I hold my power.

Teasel is a tall-growing bi-annual with sharp leaves and flower heads that were once used to tease wool for spinning. The leaves hold rainwater that was once used as an eyewash. It has a long time use in the Chinese pharmaco-poeia to treat bone ailments The tinc-ture of the root of this plant is used today as a remedy for Lyme's disease.

Indications: Is tired, weak, depleted, emotionally exhausted, confused, lost, dissatisfied; is in a toxic relationship; is codependent, abused, taken advantage of; wastes time; is on the wrong path; is constantly in disagreements; is at odds with the world.

Teasel helps a number of conditions that result in an energy loss. This is especially true of emotional conditions that deplete the energy. This can be grief or anger that is recent, intense and drains energy suddenly and dramati-cally, or it can be a long-standing obsessive grudge that brings energy down less noticeably.

The most common use for teasel is to heal conditions of energy loss due to fighting and arguments. Arguments and discord, especially when the difficul-ties remain unresolved, can cause serious disruptions to the energy flow. One can feel tired, weak and depleted. It is as if the fighting has caused a tear in the auric field that will now not hold energy. Teasel helps to rebalance these condi-tions of energy loss due to emotional trauma.

Teasel also helps energy shortages or leaks in a variety of conditions. For instance, a person may lose energy by trying too hard in a task or by over-giv-ing in relationship. In each case, the energy return is less than the energy out-put. The lesson of Teasel is to learn to use energy in a balanced and judicious manner.

Another lesson of Teasel is to be living and working in one's right livelihood. When one's work does not resonate with the soul, then energy is not being restored and the "container" weakens. Teasel helps one find the way back to living in harmony with one's soul.

At times, after taking Teasel, a person may feel solitary or withdrawn. This is a natural part of the process. There is a space created both for the replenishment of energy and for reflection on how to change one's behavior or relationships or parts of one's life that cause the energy to lower. For many of us, this is not a conscious process. Instead, we gravitate towards distractions when we are not feeling energy. Teasel brings those areas that need consideration into focus, so that the process is clear and conscious.

Energetically, Teasel repairs tears in the energy centers. These tears are caused by a variety of conditions from physical to emotional to psychic. The key symptom to all conditions is energy loss, aches and pains such as in Lyme's disease. Although Teasel flower essence is not recommended as a medical treatment for this disease, it is suggested as a useful complement.

Teasel is a wonderful essence to use for relationship counseling. It can help break patterns of abuse and victimization. It can help couples discover how to balance the flow of energy between them so that one individual is not feeling used or taken advantage of.

Teasel is useful for children who tend to be overactive and then collapse from exhaustion. It is useful for animals that become depressed when there is intense fighting or arguing in the household, or for animals who display symptoms of shock after an injury or trauma.

Preparation and Dosage: One drop of the stock essence per hundred in a dosage bottle for animals and children. Three drops per hundred for adults. When treating physical symptoms use the stock concentration.

See Also: Onion, Milk Thistle, Bull Thistle, Scarlet Pimpernel, Fraxinella.

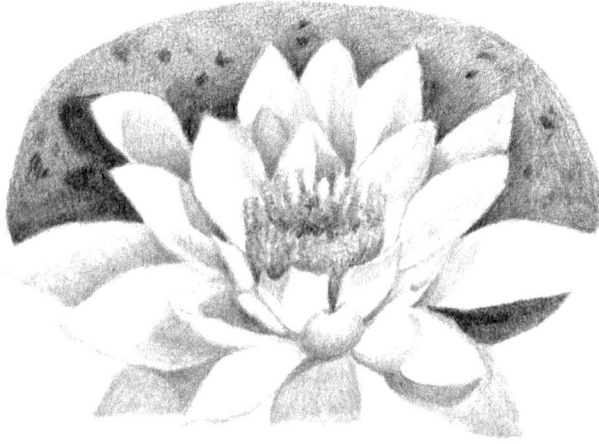

WATER LILY

Nymphaea odorata

I am filled.

Water Lily, also known as White Pond Lily is a white lotus-like flower which grows on still ponds from late spring to mid summer. Herbal preparations are used to treat deficient kidney "yin" or low fluids in the kidneys. Early allopaths used a poultice from the root to treat boils and painful tumors. In both these cases, the plant draws out the heat of the inflammation, easing pain. There are further similar treatments to the bladder, bowels and prostate, all involving the relation between heat and fluids. These treatments become significant metaphors when we begin to talk about the action of the flower essence.

Indications: Water Lily is a powerful remedy for a needy personality. This is someone who, because of a mistreatment or neglect in childhood, feels generally unfulfilled and constantly needs the attention of others. There is a wide spectrum of neediness from attention-seeking to narcissism. In all cases, the personality makes up for the lack of development by drawing energy from others.

There is an active and passive range of this imbalance in the personality. Some will create drama to receive the attention that the personality craves, while others will tend to withdraw, subconsciously aware of the attention they receive from this passive activity.

For these conditions, Water Lily creates a sense of self-sufficiency and fulfillment, giving individuals the ability to make healthier choices in their relationships.

Energetically, the second chakra is the watery domain of emotions. A safe, loving childhood produces a tremendous reservoir of energy in this area. This energy is the substance of self-esteem and is drawn up into the third chakra and projected out as confidence, will forces or active intelligence. Lack of love, lack of understanding or acceptance of an individual by primary caregivers, and later by friends, depletes the watery potential of this chakra. In most cases, it is fire in the personality that attempts to make up for the difference. A person over-uses the third chakra to make up for the feeling of lack in the second, but without the cooler etheric fluids to supply it. He or she simply does not know how to receive unconditional affection or attention, but rather learns conscious and subconscious ways of scheming, controlling and manipulating to feel a replica of a sense of fulfillment.

This is a person who may always seem at odds with someone or something. Sometimes this energy is directed at groups or takes on social or political issues. The result is the same. The intense fire in the personality converts to drama. The person takes a platform or soapbox or microphone to get attention from others.

The balance of the water and fire in these two chakras is also pivotal in maintaining healthy fluids in the system. Dryness, heat or inflammations are characteristic physical imbalances. The kidneys, pelvic area, and urinary tract are particularly susceptible to infections, cysts or boils. The fluids congesting to ease the problems are frequently too hot and cause further pain, discomfort or complications.

This essence is helpful for infants who must be left in day care most days of the week and for small children who must deal with being replaced as the youngest when another baby is born into the family. It is helpful for pets who are needy and crave attention.

Preparation and Dosage: One drop of the stock essence per 100 in a dosage bottle for animals and children. Three drops per 100 for adults. Use the stock essence to treat pelvic inflammations. Take this essence in a small cup of water.

See Also: Missouri Primrose and Blue Vervain.

WHITE COLUMBINE

Aquilegia flabellata

I know myself.

Columbine is a small woodland plant that has a delicate, bird-like flower with long spurs. This white flower is a mutation of the wild pink variety. Columbine was used herbally to kill lice and other external parasites.

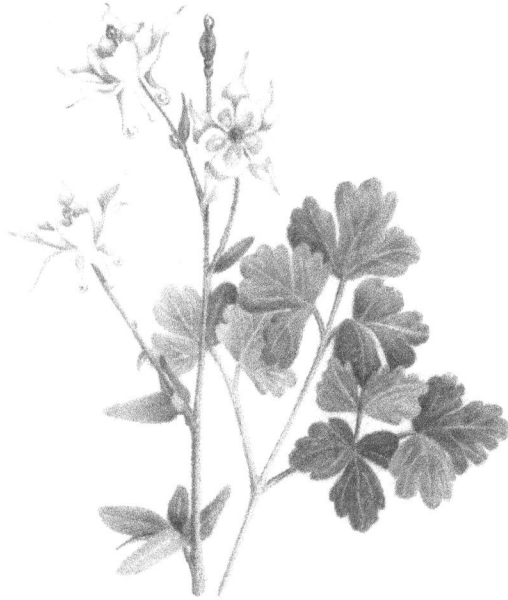

Indications: Feels lost; feels uncertain about one's own life purpose; is frustrated in searching for satisfying work; is searching for right livelihood; changes jobs often; is jealous of others; is overly ambitious; is constantly searching; fears not finding one's vocation; feels estranged; is searching for the right relationship; is overly dependent on feedback from others; has cynicism about life; has self-doubt, low self-esteem, confusion, inferiority; doesn't trust self.

White Columbine flower essence helps people who feel very lonely or confused about the direction their life is taking. There is often a feeling of something being missing or an estrangement from a feeling of purpose. This can appear as an absence of a meaningful career or a fulfilling relationship.

Although it can be true that a person has not discovered the most suitable "match" for himself or herself, White Columbine has more to do with the inner turmoil or feeling of being "lost." This feeling in the unconscious can generate confusion in the conscious mind, which in turn, creates doubt regarding choices and possibilities. It is as if there can be no career or life choice that will satisfy the longing or emptiness one feels deep in the soul.

Along with this emptiness, there can also develop other conditions: a cynicism about life, or self-doubt, or low esteem, as a result of not feeling fully connected with those things that life has presented in the form of a career or relationship; bitterness and negative attitudes that contribute to various forms of failure can arise. White Columbine can help to soothe and heal these conditions.

Sometimes people who need White Columbine flower essence have been overshadowed by very successful parents or siblings, or it can be that imprints of a past life filled with luster, success or a satisfying partnership are interfering with the present incarnation. Columbine provides a type of angelic reassurance that "all is well" and unfolding in life. Feelings of inferiority, insecurity, confusion and turmoil yield to a quiet strength and acceptance, which can cause a significant shift in success factors in the personality.

White Columbine eases the stresses that come from what a person has learned about success as he begins to compare what he perceives he has achieved against the learned values regarding success. These stresses can interfere with the natural unfolding of one's life, which may not fit with the learned program. Easing these stresses allows for more powerful manifestation of events by the soul, rather than the skewed energy of the mind, which is projecting desires and fears. The steady energy of "right purpose" accelerates the orchestration of coincidental events leading one into a satisfying career.

Energetically, the third chakra harmonizes with the upper chakras. The identity question "who am I" is given added energy. This initially clears the third chakra of confusion and the influence of the left-brain. This will temporarily suspend feelings of doubt and hesitation about meaning and purpose, giving added certainty, ease and potential movement.

Use Columbine to help those who have ended one phase of their life and are exploring other possibilities for lifestyle or career. It is helpful for those exploring the possibility of a more spiritual "vocation." It is also useful in cases of extreme ambivalence over a choice between two different careers or life-changing options.

Children who seem excessively jealous of others can benefit from White Columbine. Animals who are nervous or agitated over the absence of a companion pet that has recently died will appear calmer with the use of this essence.

Preparation and Dosage: Add one drop of stock essence to 100 drops of neutral solution. Take a few drops of this 2-3 times a day.

See Also: Lovage, Borage, Marshmallow, Golden Amaranthus, Blue Vervain, Elecampagne.

WOOD BETONY

Stachys officinalis

I am inspired.

Wood Betony is a low to medium growing plant, at home in the woodlands, gardens and meadows. It has low-growing leaves supporting a long slender stem and clusters of small purple flowers. Historically the herb has been used for many disorders from snake-bites to stomach ailments. Today it is an herbal remedy for the digestive system as well as a tonic for the brain and nervous system. Some herbalists prescribe it for enhancing memory.

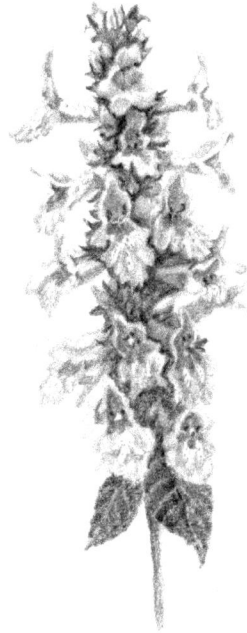

Indications: Feels unable to change behavior; feels stuck; feels uninspired; judges or condemns self; is cynical about ability of self and others to change; feels limited by nature; has frustrated idealism; feels unexpressed; feels conflicted about sexuality; feels that right and wrong are subjective and arbitrary; has trouble controlling some behaviors; feels ungrounded; feels trapped by desires.

This essence stimulates the higher functioning of the psyche. This means that a person wishing to solve a problem or issue has access to clearer aspects of thinking and awareness. It also means that a person wrestling with issues that involve higher and lower aspects of the psyche can receive additional assistance. Further, it can help artists, scientists, inventors, writers and philosophers receive the benefit of more inspired thinking.

Conflict between higher and lower natures is one of the common denominators of human existence. We struggle constantly between what we desire and what we know is best both for ourselves and in our relationship with others and the world in general. The stimulation of the higher brain functioning gives the lower nature less control over a situation; there is less struggle and therefore more choice to allow the higher reasoning to guide the individual in a situation. There is, in fact, rather than struggle, more a feeling of peace and certainty that a person is acting in integrity. Self-judgments, feelings of shame and self-condemnation are eased as a person feels less and less trapped and controlled by desires that do not align with his or her self-concept.

In addition, Wood Betony stimulates a feeling of clarity regarding the self and its expression in the world. This can be seen in the way the flower blooms, as though trumpeting something important in all directions. In fact, it is the expression of the real self that further moves the blockage or resistance of the lower chakras and helps a person feel clarity and success.

This essence can be a valuable tool to use in any type of therapy involving behavior change or modification. However, for this essence to be effective, the person must be willing or attempting to make change. It is within the crucible of the day-to-day struggle that this essence presents itself as an agent for support and deep change.

Energetically, there is a mild stimulation of the crown chakra which, in turn, stimulates the pineal gland. This enhances the higher functioning of the brain. This also makes energy more available to uplift the frequency of the lower three chakras, giving the lower nature a greater opportunity to evolve.

This is a good essence for child development in general between the ages of 4 and 7 when the child begins to learn about family values and again between ages 12 and 17 as the young person makes choices outside of the family influence. It is also good for those children who have some difficulty controlling urges and impulses or seeing the benefit in cultivating behaviors that are moderate or acceptable. This includes acting out, tantrums or inappropriate social behaviors.

This essence helps dogs and cats after neutering and can relieve tendencies to overeat in horses, cats, dogs, and ferrets.

Preparation and Dosage: Add one drop of stock essence per hundred drops of neutral solution for adults who are working on behavior change. Add one drop per three hundred for those using the essence for increased inspiration; one drop per three hundred for young children or animals and one drop per hundred for adolescents.

See also: Star Jasmine, Golden Amaranthus, Pink Amaranthus, Borage, Jack-in-the-pulpit, Pink Lady's Slipper.

WORMWOOD

Artemnesia absinthium

I release the past and
am restored.

Wormwood is a small to medium height
herb with grey-green leaves and small
yellow flowers. Its aromatic leaves are
used for "dream pillows" and as a tea
for internal cleansing and restoration of
the stomach and colon. It has also been
used to rid the system of parasites and was an addi-
tive to the European liquor, absinthe. This liquor was
eventually made illegal in several countries because of its
addictive nature and because of a kind of dementia that
resulted from its continued use.

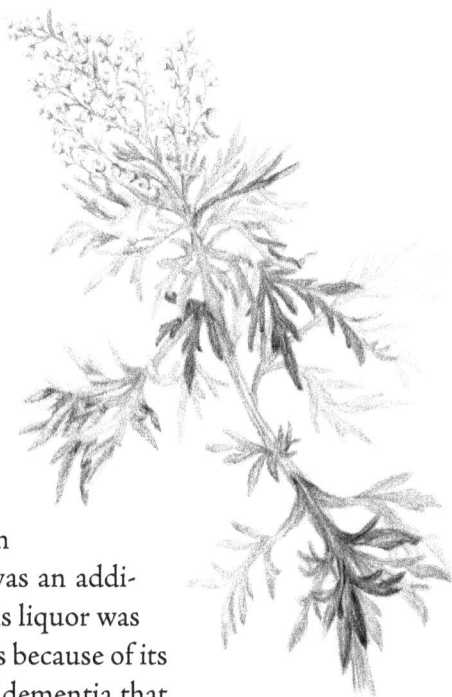

Indications: Can't get over an incident or relationship; obsesses; feels fated or
doomed; has unwanted thoughts or feelings; is exhausted; burnt-out, stuck in
old habits; feels addicted; has bad luck; feels caught in the past; can't end relationships; feels unable to enjoy the present.

Wormwood flower essence is advisable in conditions of lingering negative
or unwanted thoughts, feelings or habits. This usually means that someone has
done some work on an issue but some parts of it remain in the psyche. For
instance one may have worked to end a relationship but cannot stop thinking
about the person. Or one may be bothered by feelings one has towards another
long after a relationship has ended. Wormwood clears out the psychic "debris"
that remains in the energy field, even when one has done some processing or
therapeutic work.

Sometimes a person who is attempting to change a habit or a behavior will
at first experience initial or partial success, but then regresses into the old
behavior. Many of our habits have an "emotional core" somewhere in the
psyche that needs to be released before there is the possibility for more complete freedom from the issue. Here Wormwood provides a useful complement
to other programs of behavior change, but it is more effective if the person

receives some additional support for the emotions that may surface during the treatment period.

Wormwood helps the thinking process become clearer. It does this by releasing the deeper imprints in the subconscious, which often distort thoughts as they surface. With Wormwood, thoughts surface more quickly about how things really are or insights about what must be done can be more easily accessed.

Wormwood is an ideal essence for people who have had very difficult lives. These are long-term survivors who have been successful in attaining a level of health, balance, and happiness, but who have scars to show for it. With Wormwood, there is a feeling of rebirth or restoration that helps a person to understand their lessons more deeply, and to embrace their lives and existence rather than feel some level or regret, self-pity or negativity.

Energetically, there is a cleansing process which begins as the third chakra reverses its spin. Chakra two, in turn, reverses its general pull upward and begins to empty debris that the personality no longer needs to hold. It is here through chakra two that all releasing of toxic emotions occurs.

Use Wormwood when retraining animals who have acquired bad habits, or with children who are unusually resistant to making change in their daily schedules. Use also with children who continually bring up specific bothersome events or times in the past.

Preparation and Dosage: One drop of the stock essence per 100 for animals and children. Three drops per 100 for adults.

See Also: Milk Thistle, Canada Thistle.

Repertory

ABANDONMENT

Black Currant – For feelings of abandonment; for deep fears related to identity shifts and crises. Eases the pain of abandonment and vulnerability to fears that threaten the experience of the self.

Butterfly Weed – Helps adults who have difficulty committing to relationships because of childhood abandonment issues.

Gravel Root – For fear of being left alone. Eases this fear, allowing a person to gradually accept and benefit from periods of solace.

Stinging Nettle – For releasing pain and grief related to partings and endings; for healing deep hurt from abandonment.

ABUNDANCE

Hyssop – For fear of pleasure; for self-sabotage. Helps undo some of the irrational foothold of judgment and self-condemnation, which in turn eases guilt and shame-based patterns.

Golden Amaranthus – Helps a person be in the flow of abundance.

Missouri Primrose – Awakens worthiness, increasing a person's ability to manifest abundance.

Teasel – Helps a person receive and keep energy, making manifestation of abundance possible.

ABUSE

Back Cohosh – For those attracted to dark personalities who continue cycles of abuse. Provides clarity, lifting the spell and showing other people and situations for what they are and not what they pretend to be.

Blackberry Lily – For treating sexual abuse. Releases sexual trauma.

Canada Thistle – For treating abuse that was family inflicted. Helps soften and dislodge hardened beliefs, attitudes and feelings in the personality directed towards some aspect of family or community membership.

Missouri Primrose – For those who have neglect in their personal history. Helps one learn to accept and receive love, friendship, goodness, pleasure, and other forms of self-nurturing.

Motherwort – For those who do not know how to protect themselves from abusive personalities. Helps one set boundaries and respond if needed with constructive, assertive behavior. Balances strength and softness.

Pink Amaranthus – For the confusion of feelings of love with many of the negative emotions that surface simultaneously with an attraction to another.

Helps one to be reflective and to heal some of the deeper issues of the past relationships.

Stinging Nettle – For neglect, trauma, or abuse in childhood; for those who are often in conflict with others. Eases pain in the present that is intensified or skewed from untreated early childhood pain. Helps one become more aware of the basis of irrational responses rather than degenerating to externalizing and blaming.

Teasel – For abuse resulting in patterns of energy victimization. Helps one discover how to balance the exchange of energy with others. For those who are repeatedly taken advantage of.

ACCIDENT-PRONE

Potato – For the accident-prone. Anchors the self on the earth plane as one expands, awakens, and develops.

Water Lily – For those who attract drama; for over-reliance on acting out extreme emotional states in order to exercise control. Offers a sense of self-sufficiency, fulfillment, and emotional ease.

ADDICTION (SEE ALSO "RELEASE," "GROUNDING," "SELF-ESTEEM")

Black Currant – For an increase in addictive behavior when ideas of self or reality are challenged.

Blackberry Lily – For sexual addictions. Releases repressed sexual trauma.

Blue Vervain – For addictions that calm the nerves; for addictions of a high stress life; for self-neglect addictions. Provides a soothing energy, making it easier to access emotions that are being shut out of the system.

Comfrey – Helps one treat addictions by going deeper into the therapeutic process.

Fraxinella – For those who feel stuck, unable to cope with life, tend to repress feelings or memories. Energies of frustration are released and replaced with positive feelings towards success, as well as new ideas and possibilities that have not previously been considered.

Hyssop – For guilt addiction or guilt-based addictions.

Indian Tobacco – For assistance in tobacco addictions. Keeps balance in the mental body.

Missouri Primrose – For eating disorders and other addictive behaviors based on low self-esteem. Helps one develop self-nurturing behaviors.

Marshmallow – For those in 12-step programs, who are working on accessing their feelings; softens the entire emotional system so that emotions can be accessed, expressed, and released.

Potato – For those who, in seeking an expanded or spiritual life, are attracted exclusively to things that produce a "high." Gently brings the person back into the body, into a less expanded reality where he or she can be more in touch with physical and emotional issues.

Stinging Nettle – For addiction to alcohol or drugs related to untreated early childhood pain. Helps one become more aware of the sources of one's addictions and begin working with the deeper personal issues rather than degenerate to externalizing and blaming.

Sumac – For those who feel like giving up, are discouraged, have lost motivation. Brings a gentle strength and stamina to the system; assists in maintaining connection with the heart during difficult phases and transitions in recovery.

Wood Betony – For those who feel unable to change or control behavior; cynical about ability of self and others to change. Stimulates higher reasoning to guide one in situations.

Wormwood – For those who feel stuck in old habits, caught in the past, or in addictive behaviors; helps to release unconscious imprints and energetic "cords."

ADOLESCENCE (SEE ALSO "CHILDREN")

Bull Thistle – A general tonic for adolescent and teenage rebelliousness.

Golden Amaranthus – For students during junior and senior years of high school and college.

Hemp Agrimony – Assists adolescents in the development of leadership qualities and social grace.

Horseradish – Benefits adolescents preparing for college and career choices, especially when there seems to be avoidance and procrastination over these issues.

Lady's Mantle – A general remedy for the oldest boy or girl in the family.

Lemon Balm – For the early adolescent stage when a child is beginning to feel anxious about the future.

Lilac – For adolescents who have poor posture and low confidence.

Lovage – Helpful for any stage of life exploration when one considers choices and the future, such as college selection during junior and senior year of high school.

Motherwort – For adolescents who have become moody, withdrawn, or combative.

Onion – For children during disappointment or loss. With adolescents, it can prevent or treat anger that can follow loss, or the death of someone close.

Pink Amaranthus – For teenagers who have poor attitudes about relationships, especially those who have parents who do not have a healthy partnership.

Pink Lady's Slipper – For adolescents who are not fitting into the framework of our educational system; for complementary treatment with any therapy or alternative educational activity exploring deeper meanings and values with young people.

Skullcap – For teenagers who often become self-absorbed, cynical, very selective and guarded about friendships. During such a period there may be an increased insensitivity to others or a general self-neglect around matters of health and safety.

Solomon's Seal – For adolescents who are inflexible or cannot cope with change or with things going wrong.

Sumac – For adolescents who do not like school. Helps sustain energy to continue working towards any goal. Also for when deciding about a long-term life investment such as a college education. Helps those who have difficulty looking and planning for the future.

Wood Betony – For development in general between ages 12 and 17 as the young person makes choices outside of the family influence. Also for adolescents who have some difficulty controlling urges and impulses, or seeing the benefit in cultivating behaviors that are moderate or acceptable.

Wormwood – For adolescents who can't get over an incident or relationship; for adolescent obsessions. Helps release unconscious imprints.

AGGRESSIVENESS – SEE "ANGER"

AGING / ELDERS

Black Currant – For fears of death and of not existing; for profound questions about life and death. Gives courage to go beyond internal fears and conflicts, and so to continue one's journey into truth, light, and meaning. Eases the fears and overwhelming dread of those who are dying and do not believe in the survival of the soul after death.

Indian Tobacco – For subconscious fears related to death and dying.

Lemon Balm – For those who are anxious about death. Offers peace and calmness when difficult emotions surface.

Marshmallow – Eases resistance to aging.

Sumac – For the onset of retirement or any major life change when there is difficulty feeling the energy to look and plan ahead. Strengthens one's foundational rhythm and the ability to sustain drive and energy.

ALIENATION – SEE "LONELINESS," "SHYNESS"

ALOOFNESS – SEE "PESSIMISM," "SOCIALNESS"

AMBITION

Blue Vervain – For those who feel obliged to live their lives as leaders, role models, or providers; for those who cannot yield to a safer, healthier, more practical approach because of pride, ambition, or role identity.

Golden Amaranthus – For leadership "personalities" who take on many tasks and responsibilities; for original, charismatic, competitive people, who are often very successful in their endeavors yet privately feel alone, misunderstood, and frustrated.

White Columbine – For those who appear overly ambitious but are constantly searching; for fears of not finding a meaningful vocation. Eases feelings of inferiority, insecurity, confusion, and turmoil.

AMBIVALENCE – SEE "CLARITY," DECISION-MAKING"

ANGER

Blue Vervain – For aggressiveness. Balances the driven personality and makes it easier to access other emotions that are being shut out of the system.

Bull Thistle – For anger towards people or institutions that one perceives as controlling. Releases negative past experiences with structure or authority. One is more able to see situations clearly and to trust healthy structures and leaders.

Canada Thistle – For unresolved anger towards family members. Softens and dislodges hardened beliefs, attitudes, and feelings in the personality that are directed towards some aspect of family or community membership.

Lady's Mantle – For those who have anger attacks. Imparts a feeling of strength and protection which supports the ability to contain and use one's own feminine energies.

Lungwort – For those who repress anger through shallow breathing; for fear of anger or annoyance over small things. Helps to move blockages and the symptoms they can intensify, so that energy flows properly in rhythm with the breath.

Marshmallow – For hardened emotions, inflexibility, holding grudges. Teaches how to soften interactions with those who we do not feel connected to; helps us to feel love when angry or hurt.

Milk Thistle – For letting go of deep anger, resentment, or other held feelings that block the flow of love; for getting in touch with repressed anger or easing an angry personality.

Onion – For the grieving process, including the initial stages where there is anger and frustration. Helps one access and process grief.

Pink Amaranthus – For those who hit or slap others; for those who have low tolerance for mistakes or shortcomings of friends or partners; for the confusion of feelings of love with negative emotions that arise out of being in love.

Motherwort – For those who attracts angry and abusive personalities; also for those who can be angry, harsh, or overbearing. Helps replace anger with healthy boundaries.

Scullcap – Helps one develop sensitivity towards those we are angry with.

Teasel – For anger that is recent, intense, and suddenly and dramatically drains energy; for energy loss due to fighting and arguments.

ANIMAL CARE

Black Cohosh – For horses, dogs, cats and birds who are at the bottom of the pecking order; also for dogs who react to loud or deep voices.

Blackberry Lily – For animals who exhibit sudden and latent antisocial behavior. (Often they have accessed a repressed imprint in someone in the household.)

Black Currant – For animals of caretakers who have a preoccupation with fears of death. Helps animals remain free from the stress and fears that surround such individuals.

Blessed Thistle – For general household stress that may be transferred to the animal, especially for animals when there is a death in the family; also gives added comfort to dying animals.

Blue Vervain – For animals who are intensely trained, such as show or racing horses and guide or guard dogs; helps animals relax more deeply during "down time," and deal better with the high stress of their jobs.

Borage – For animals who are depressed, sleep more or change eating habits in response to being left unattended for long periods. For sensitive animals who lose vigor during times of suppressed turmoil in their human family, such as when dogs or cats become lethargic when their caretakers are in a period of not speaking to each other out of anger.

Bull Thistle – Relieves stress of confinement for all animals, especially dogs bred close to ancestral strains of wolves, as well as caged birds, pet rodents, and turtles.

Canada Thistle – Helps animals who move from small to larger families, or those who may have previously been part of a large family and were mistreated or subjected to over-stressful family living. For animals (as well as humans) to heal from bone fractures and surgery.

Celandine – Enhances animal training, especially in situations where new behaviors are being introduced. There may be a noticeable enhancement of the pet's "attempts" to communicate.

Elecampagne – For animals who have been rescued or who come from abusive previous owners. The safety of the new situation and the personality of the new caretaker are internalized more quickly.

Fraxinella – For rabbits and other animals who live in confinement, especially when they are prone to cysts, infections, and blockages in the system.

Golden Amaranthus – For animals who have terminal illness. In some cases there can be an easing of the symptoms of the disease; in others there is assistance in making the experience of passing peaceful, dignified, and sacred. Also for human family members of an animal who may be close to death but is hanging on in spite of many challenging symptoms.

Habenaro Pepper – For rescued animals whose reflex behaviors were likely acquired from previous abusive owners – such as when a certain type of voice, tone, or behavior like picking up a stick, for instance, causes the animal to cower or become aggressive.

Hemp Agrimony – For animals and caged birds that are antisocial or very territorial. For animals who are bred to protect or be on guard; who have difficulty letting down their guard with other animals or humans. Helps animals feel their own natural curiosities and connections to others.

Hyssop – For animals trained through traditional methods involving physical punishment, especially when the punishment is inconsistent and sometimes harsh. Also for animals subjected to trainings that are different from the beliefs and personality of the primary caretaker.

Horseradish – For animals who become depressed and inactive in response to their caretaker's emotions, or express "bad temper" during stressful times. For animals who tend to have poor circulation, slow digestion, or colds.

Indian Pipe – For animals who change caretakers, for animals who require a lot of affection, for pound animals and most caged birds.

Jack-in-the-pulpit – For animals who are having difficulty integrating their instincts with their environment. For all caged or confined animals who begin to display self-destructive or compulsive behaviors; for neutered animals, animals who overeat and animals who do not sleep well.

Japanese Knotweed – Shortens adaptation time when a new animal joins a family, especially when other animals are already present in the home. Relieves growing pains and stresses.

Lady's Mantle – For overly aggressive or antisocial animals and pets immediately after being neutered.

Lilac – Promotes better relaxation for many types of dogs who feel a responsibility to protect or perform.

Lovage – For more docile or timid animals or those low in the pecking order. Offers feelings of contentment, security, and strength.

Lemon Balm – For periods when animals are restless and sleepless. Helpful after an animal experiences an incident of high stress requiring the release of adrenalin. Show dogs and horses will benefit from a single dosage both before and after their performance.

Lilac – Promotes better relaxation for many types of dogs who feel a responsibility to protect or to perform.

Lobelia – For animals who have been punished for being noisy. Provides a release of the stress from repressing an otherwise natural instinct. Also for when an animal seems to be attempting to communicate something new, which is sometimes the case when new behaviors appear for no apparent reason.

Lungwort – For timid or shy animals, or those who are low in the pecking order.

Marshmallow – A complement to retraining animals to be less structured or on guard, or when trying to break any previous excessive conditioning, including "retired" animals such as: show animals, police dogs, racehorses or greyhounds. Helps these animals relax and attune to new, less rigid trainers or masters. Also for hardening of tissue in animals.

Milk Thistle – For any animal who has suffered abuse in the past, which includes most all rescued animals and those bought in pet stores.

Missouri Primrose – For domesticated feral cats or animals who were starved by their owners. For any animals who tend to eat too much.

Motherwort – For animals who are very territorial or timid and fearful.

Onion – For animals who have been mistreated, especially those who tend to whine for no apparent reason; for animals in the households of grieving family members.

Pink Amaranthus – For animals who have been abused or abandoned and are relearning to trust a new owner, especially dogs who have very affectionate natures.

Pink Lady's Slipper – A strongly beneficial tonic for all household, caged, or shelter animals, improving both temperament and physical functioning.

Potato – For reintroducing a wild animal back into nature.

Scarlet Pimpernel – For animals who have lost a companion pet or are sullen, lethargic, or depressed; for rescued animals who have a susceptibility to rashes or inflammations.

Skullcap – For animals who occasionally lash out at their caregivers or others without apparent cause.

Stinging Nettle – For animals from shelters or those who have been punished or beaten.

Star Jasmine – For all pets who experience a lethargy or depression, especially larger animals (such as large dogs, horses, and many wild animals in captivity) as these tend to feel their own weight as part of a lower mood.

Teasel – For animals who become depressed when there is intense fighting or arguing in the household; for animals who display symptoms of shock after an injury or trauma.

Sumac – A general tonic for animals entering old age. Especially useful for animals who are "retired," or no longer able to keep up some of their previous routines with their caregivers.

Water Lily – For pets who are needy and crave attention.

White Columbine. – Calms animals who are nervous or agitated over the absence of a companion pet that has recently passed away.

Wood Betony – For dogs and cats after neutering. Can relieve tendencies to over-eat in horses, cats, dogs, and ferrets.

Wormwood – For retraining animals who have acquired bad habits.

ANXIETY

Blue Vervain – For mental stress; for anxiety due to overwork or feeling the obligation to live their lives as leaders, role models, or providers; for those who have inability to relax. Balances a driven personality.

Bull Thistle – For fears and anxiety about authorities and being controlled by others. Assists in releasing negative past experiences with structure or authority. One is more able to see situations clearly and to trust healthy structures and leaders.

Butterfly Weed – For those who feel anxiety over commitment.

Lemon Balm – For mental turbulence. Produces calmness, which allows deeper emotional exploration. One's mind is able to remain keen while enveloped by peacefulness.

Gravel Root – For anxiety over friendships and relationships. Eases fears of being alone. Offers a steadiness and confidence to venture out on one's own. Helps one gradually accept and benefit from periods of solace.

Lungwort – For those who lose their breath in anxious moments. Helps to move blockages, and the symptoms they can intensify, so energy flows properly in rhythm with the breath.

Pink Amaranthus – For those who feel anxious when in love.

Scarlet Pimpernel – For many aspects of difficult emotions such as obsession, anxiety. and fear. Helps one understand and transform intense emotions and release blocked energy in the heart.

ARROGANCE

Blessed Thistle – For agnostic or atheist personalities. For those who attracts over-bearing, arrogant personality types. Helps ease a fear of life or of the Powers that guide all things.

Blue Vervain – For strong, dominating or arrogant personalities. Balances a driven personality. Helps develop ease and versatility.

Black Cohosh – For fear of strong, arrogant personalities.

Golden Amaranthus – For those who cannot rely on others. For leaders who go against the tide. Helps one relax and let go of over-control.

Solomon's Seal – For those who are not willing to change. Eases and softens extreme pride, arrogance, or willfulness. Helps one develop alternatives.

Japanese Knotweed – For those who cannot work in teams. Enhances sensitivity and ability to work together in groups.

Marshmallow – For "hard" personalities. Softens arrogance.

APATHY – SEE "ENGAGEMENT WITH LIFE," "PESSIMISM," "STAGNATION"

ATHLETICS

Comfrey – For co-ordination, muscle education, and control.

Sumac – For endurance and stamina.

Lungwort – For developing breathing capacity.

AUTHORITY – SEE ALSO "LEADERSHIP," "POWER"

AVOIDANCE – SEE "RESISTANCE"

AWARENESS (SEE ALSO "INTUITION," "PEACE")

Celandine – For communication blocks and misunderstandings; for self–expression, receiving inspiration or higher thoughts. Enhances many aspects of communication.

Fraxinella – For those who tend to repress feelings or memories; for those who cannot get past or resolve an issue. Releases frustration, often offering insight, new ideas, and possibilities that have not previously been considered.

Golden Amaranthus – Offers the deeply held "knowledge" that we are protected and guided on the highest level, giving one permission to let the guard down, to trust, to enjoy, to go with the flow, to "let go and let God."

Habanero Pepper – Holds one in connection to the physical while doing emotional work; prevents separation, drifting; promotes clarity and presence, at the same time helps to bring movement to repressed feelings.

Hemp Agrimony – For those who have a fear, memory, or feeling that it is unsafe to be with others, and so have many social fears. Assists in the release of such imprints, which prevent the feeling of connection. Opens one to awareness of the interconnectedness of all things through the heart.

Indian Pipe – Expands awareness of the presence of universal love. Develops a sensitivity and receptivity to a higher love vibration; seeing and feeling the love in every moment.

Jack-in-the-pulpit – Enhances the awareness of and relationship to one's inner voice.

Japanese Knotweed – Enhances group awareness, sensitivity, and telepathy. Provides energy, calmness and insight.

Lemon Balm – Produces a calm that allows deeper emotional exploration. One's mind remains keen while enveloped by peacefulness.

Scarlet Pimpernel – Helps one understand and transform intense emotions such as obsession, anxiety, and fear.

Skullcap – Increases awareness of one's intuitive response to others; helps one to feel and know another from the other's perspective; enhances empathy in the healing process.

BEAUTY – SEE ALSO "INSPIRATION"

Elecampagne – For times when new feelings, talents, insights are awakened. Helps one identify more deeply with newly discovered power and beauty in one's self. Balances and integrates new experiences of spirituality.

Indian Pipe – For stages when one feels unloved. Expands awareness of the presence of universal love, seeing and feeling the love in every moment.

Pink Lady's Slipper – Helps one realize the beauty and subtle power of the earth and human nature.

BLAME – SEE "SHAME"

BOUNDARIES – SEE "PROTECTION"

BROKEN-HEARTEDNESS (SEE ALSO "ROMANTIC LOVE")

Butterfly Weed – For those who cannot commit to long-term relationships; for fear and sadness when initial stages of "being in love" shift. Eases fears of being hurt or trapped, allowing for more maturity and deeper relationships.

Borage – For those who become downcast or discouraged after a breakup. Offers hope and soothes the heart.

Pink Amaranthus – For those who experience patterns of failure in relationships. Helps one become aware of and utilize the positive love energies that are available rather than focusing on fears, doubts and negativity. Helps one feel safe in opening to love.

Fraxinella – For recent trauma and "broken-hearts." Keeps the energies of hurt and pain from sinking into the subconscious; Also for the final stages of healing a trauma. Releases hurt and frustration, and redirects energies.

Wormwood – For those who can't get over a relationship; feeling unable to enjoy the present. Moves out old patterns that have attached to the heart; releases, breaks, and removes unconscious imprints and energetic "cords."

'BURN-OUT" – SEE "EXHAUSTION"

CALMNESS – SEE "PEACEFULNESS," "EASE OF LIFE"

CERTAINTY (SEE ALSO "CLARITY," "CONFIDENCE")

Blessed Thistle – For certainty about God's loving presence.

Celandine – For certainty in all aspects of communication.

Comfrey – For certainty and clarity about painful memories.

Indian Tobacco – For certainty of goodness and love on the path of spiritual development.

Indian Pipe – For certainty in the presence of love.

Lobelia – For certainty in self-expression.

Motherwort – Becoming certain about appropriate responses towards threatening personalities.

White Columbine – For certainty regarding life choices and professional identity.

CHANGE – SEE "TRANSFORMATION"

CHILDREN (SEE ALSO "ADOLESCENCE")

Black Cohosh – For children who are afraid of loud or strong personalities. This might be men with deep voices or women with high shrill voices. Also for children with fears of people who are wearing certain hats or uniforms.

Blackberry Lily – Preschool children who express strong instinctive dislikes for certain other children can benefit from this essence. Useful for past life work when some event from another lifetime is interfering with relationships in the present incarnation.

Blessed Thistle – For children during times when their developing minds come to grips with some of the deeper questions about the existence and nature of God. It is best here if the parent or caregiver takes the essence too for a day or two, while the questions and the answers are alive in the soul of the child.

Blue Vervain – For firstborn children, high-achieving children or children of high-achieving parents. Helps them to deal better with daily stresses.

Borage – For grammar school-aged children who do not like school, either because they are afraid of school, or because they become bored and apathetic because of the monotony and repetition.

Bull Thistle – For children who excessively challenge or rebel against rules, authority, and schedules.

Butterfly Weed – For children who are generally dependent and needy. Helps with resistance to toilet training, especially when a new baby is born into the family just before or during the training period. Helpful during family therapy, especially in the early stages.

Celandine – For children who have difficulty speaking, being understood, and understanding others.

Comfrey – For students studying for tests; for athletes seeking better performance in sports, especially where reflex and coordination are key factors in success.

Elecampagne – For broad applications to childhood by providing a new level of self-acceptance. Helps with the stress older children feel when a newborn replaces them as the youngest. Helps younger children with the stress of measuring up to standards set by older children. Also helps extreme competition between siblings.

Fraxinalla – For children who tend to hold grudges or those who are easily frustrated by failure. It can help balance both of these conditions, helping the child stay away from identities and attitudes that might hold the patterns within the personality.

Gravel Root – For anti-social, lonely children, who do not feel connected to others.

Golden Amaranthus – For hardworking success-oriented children.

Habanero Pepper – For children who had any kind of complication, difficulty or trauma in the birthing process and later develop difficulties such as forgetfulness, absent mindedness or inability to focus.

Hemp Agrimony – Help ease selfishness and extreme independence in children.

Horseradish – Benefits children who tend to be timid and lack confidence.

Hyssop – For children who obsessively fear punishment.

Indian Pipe – For children who do not feel loved. For children who, while often having loving parents, must deal regularly with adults or siblings who are not loving or affectionate, as with children who feel picked on by other children or siblings, or children with stern teachers.

Indian Tobacco – For children who have genuine spiritual experiences but have begun to fear or bury them. Helps the child to co-exist easily with spiritual gifts or experiences, and not push them into the subconscious because of fear.

Jack-In-the-pulpit – For children who ask many questions about deeper aspects of life and death.

Japanese Knotweed – Helpful for children when a new baby comes into the family. Helps changes in status and roles to happen more smoothly.

Lady's Mantle – For children beginning to socialize. A good general remedy for the oldest boy or girl in the family.

Lemon Balm – For children who are unable to relax or slow down or who become tired easily.

Lilac – For overly independent or responsible children, or those who seem to fear accepting responsibility. Helps develop a healthy balance between self-reliance and reliance on others.

Lobelia – For children who are late talkers or those who have a problem with stuttering, especially if it is stress related.

Lovage – For children when they begin school, change schools, or move to a new home; also helpful for any stage of life exploration when one considers choices and the future.

Lungwort – For very shy or sensitive children.

Marshmallow – For children who tend to have difficulty letting go of hurt, anger, or criticism.

Milk Thistle – For adopted children who are physically abusive or who cannot control their anger; for children who are prone to violence; for dislike of sibling(s).

Missouri Primrose – For the oldest child, especially when they take on adult responsibilities early; also for any child who tends to take studying and preparing for the future too seriously.

Motherwort – For the oldest child of each gender in any family; for children who have lost one or both parents.

Onion – For children during disappointment or loss. Prevents unconscious fears of death and loss from lodging in the personality. With older children, it can prevent or treat the acting out of anger that can follow loss or the death of someone close; for children who tend to be very emotional.

Pink Amaranthus – For children who have difficulty making friends.

Pink Lady's Slipper – For children who don't fit into the framework of our educational system; for complementary treatment with any therapy or alternative educational activity exploring deeper meanings and values with young people.

Potato – For children who are very imaginative and sometimes become confused about what is real, or they prefer to stay in their imaginations for undue periods of time; for gifted children who develop a talent or a strong intellect at a rapid pace. Helps a child keep a healthy foundation and perspective, so that their development can proceed in a balanced way.

Scarlet Pimpernel – For children who are withdrawn or who tend towards sulking. Helps, with some professional guidance, promote better communication with them.

Skullcap – For small children who are very inward and strike out unexpectedly at others.

Solomon's Seal – For children who become frustrated easily when things change or go wrong. Helps one let go of control or attachment to outcomes, and learn to refocus and adapt to mishaps.

Star Jasmine – For very serious, responsible, or mature children. Helps maintain their childlike, joyful nature.

Stinging Nettle – For adopted children, children from broken homes, and children whose parents are going through separation and divorce. Eases emotional pain.

Sumac – For children who resist schoolwork or other work geared towards long-term goals. Helps a child "feel" the value of their work even when the physical or social impact might not be readily observable.

Teasel – For children who tend to be overactive and then collapse from exhaustion. Helps one learn to use energy in a balanced and judicious manner.

Water Lily – For infants who must be left in day-care most days of the week; for small children who must deal with being replaced as the youngest when another baby is born into the family.

White Columbine – For children who seem excessively jealous of others.

Wood Betony – For child development in general between the ages of 4 and 7, when the child begins to learn about family values. Also for children who have some difficulty controlling urges and impulses, including acting out, tantrums, or inappropriate social behaviors, or have difficulty seeing the benefit in cultivating behaviors that are moderate or acceptable.

Wormwood – For children who are unusually resistant to making change in their daily schedules; for children who continually bring up specific bothersome events or times in the past.

CLARITY (SEE ALSO AWARENESS)

Black Cohosh – For gaining clarity into victimization. Helps one understand situations for what they are and not what they pretend to be.

Black Currant – For inability to focus on daily matters when ideas of self and reality are challenged. Gives courage and illumination to look at and integrate the new experience and the new meaning of "self" that the experience carries.

Celandine – For communication blocks and misunderstandings; self-expression. Enhances communication and the reception of inspiration or higher thoughts.

Habanero Pepper – For mental fogginess, separation, or drifting. Promotes clarity, presence, and connection to the physical, while at the same time it stimulates movement of repressed feelings.

Jack-in-the-pulpit – For difficulty coordinating one's spiritual impulses and their expression in the world. Also for exploration of new forms of spiritual thought; for difficulty expressing philosophical or spiritual ideas. Strengthens one's relationship to one's inner voice, making the clear expression of authentic spirituality more possible.

Japanese Knotweed – For groups seeking clarity. Enhances group awareness, sensitivity, and telepathy; provides energy, calmness and insight.

Lemon Balm – For clarity and calmness in emotional or stressful times. Helps one's mind remain keen while enveloped by peacefulness, allowing deeper emotional exploration.

Potato – For dreamy, escapist fantasies or delusional thinking. Gently brings one back into the body, into "normal reality" where one can reflect about the experience, integrate it, and then act.

Star Jasmine – For those who cannot think clearly. Adds clarity to intellectual pursuits and increases insight and illumination to areas where the intellect receives inspiration from the intuition.

White Columbine – For those who feel uncertain or lost in life choices. Provides insight into true identity and highest purpose.

Wood Betony – Stimulates a feeling of clarity regarding the self and its expression in the world. Also for those wrestling with controlling their desires. Stimulates higher reasoning to guide the individual in a situation.

Wormwood – For unwanted thoughts or feelings, Helps the thinking process become clearer by releasing the deeper imprints in the subconscious, which often distort thoughts as they surface.

CO-DEPENDENCE – SEE "DEPENDENCE"

COMMUNICATION

Blue Vervain – Helps driven people become more receptive to input.

Celandine – For enhancing self-expression, receiving inspiration or higher thoughts; for communication blocks and misunderstandings. Enhances many aspects of communication.

Jack-in-the-pulpit – For those who feel unable to express what they feel to be true, are unclear and unwilling to dialogue about beliefs; for thoughtful people who feel as if they know something but cannot fully express it. Strengthens one's relationship to one's inner voice.

Japanese Knotweed – For the enhancement of group communication, sensitivity, and telepathy.

Lobelia – For many difficulties related to speaking. For lecturers, singers, and teachers; students learning about public speaking; for those who keep silent in groups, feeling uncertain what to say. Offers courage to express and speak the truth regarding one's self.

Missouri Primrose – For those who are shy or inexpressive of their own truths. Helps one develop self-esteem and the ability to recognize or utilize one's own power.

Pink Lady's Slipper – For gifted people who have trouble fitting in or expressing the awareness they hold within. Helps one realize the beauty of one's being, as well as its subtle power, making it more available to the conscious mind for expression.

Potato – For those who avoid getting to the point; for nervous people who talk obsessively. Gently brings one back into the "body" where one can reflect about experience, integrate it and then express it in a practical manner.

Teasel – For those who lose energy interacting with others, including acting out, tantrums, or inappropriate social behaviors. Renews and rebalances one's energy. Helps one learn to use energy in a balanced and judicious manner.

CONCENTRATION – SEE "CLARITY," "STUDY / SCHOOLWORK"

CONFIDENCE (SEE ALSO   "POWER," "MANIFESTATION," "SELF-ESTEEM," "SELF-EXPRESSION")

Celandine – For confidence related to being understood and understanding others.

Lilac – Helps a general attitude of apparent "laziness," especially when due to lack of confidence or fear.

Lovage – For confidence in taking action; moving into the world with a sense of safety and joy; developing a sense of exhilaration in walking one's path.

Elecampagne – For those who identify with negative aspects of their personality; helps one transition into a new identity, leaving old, negative imprints behind.

Jack-in-the-pulpit – For lack of confidence and lack of expression of one's inner ideas and feelings. Strengthens one's relationship to one's inner voice.

Lady's Mantle – For those who do not feel confident, who can't feel their self apart from others. Imparts a feeling of strength and protection that supports one's ability to contain and to use power.

Missouri Primrose – For lack of confidence and low self-esteem. Helps one accept and receive love, friendship, goodness, pleasure, and other forms of self-nurturing. Self-nurturing, vital energies are taken in, which are later converted into confidence and goal-directed activities.

Sumac – For times when ones has lost confidence in one's goals; the meaning for continuing seems to have gone.

White Columbine – For those who feel uncertain or lost in life choices. Provides insight into true identity and highest purpose.

CONFLICT

Black Cohosh – Addresses fear of violence and conflict; fear of strong personalities; fear of being hurt. Treats fears, helping one to be able to include a healthier range of responses to strong personalities.

Celandine – For communication blocks and misunderstandings. Enhances many aspects of communication; for self-expression; for receiving inspiration or higher thought.

Hemp Agrimony – Enhances the awareness of the interconnectedness of all things through the heart; eases feelings and perceptions of aloneness, or disconnectedness.

Golden Amaranthus – For general feelings of always being misunderstood and frustrated rather than for a particular conflict; for obsessions with past conflicts. Offers deep relief as energies of frustration are dislodged and moved out of the energy field. Allows access to creative solutions to problems.

Jack-in-the-pulpit – For those in conflict with, frustrated by, or estranged from organized spiritual or religious groups and/or leaders. Also for those whose spiritual impulses conflict with their expression in the world. Strengthens one's relationship to the inner voice, enabling the expression of an authentic spirituality. Helps resolve conflicts between past spiritual experiences and present spiritual insight.

Japanese Knotweed – Enhances group awareness, sensitivity and telepathy; provides energy, calmness and insight; enhances group experience and ceremony.

Skullcap – Increases awareness of one's intuitive response to others; helps one to feel and know another from the other's perspective; enhances empathy in the healing process.

Stinging Nettle – For those who are often in conflict with others. Helps one become aware of the basis of his or her irrational responses and begin working with the deeper personal issues rather than degenerating to externalizing and blaming. For those in emotional pain from conflicts, offenses, misunderstandings, or pain from more intense situations such as abuse or torment.

Teasel – For energy loss caused by an intense argument, for those in constant disagreements, at odds with the world. Heals energy "leaks."

CONFUSION (SEE ALSO "CLARITY," "GROUNDING")

Habanero Pepper – Alleviates several forms of mental fogginess.

Indian Tobacco – Helps to steady irrational fears or confusions. Keeps balance in the mental body during expanded states. Helps to release subconscious fears of spirituality.

Jack-in-the-pulpit – For those who are confused or in conflict with their own spiritual impulses and their day-to-day expression of spirituality in the world. Also for those exploring new forms of spiritual thought, for deep thinkers who feel as if they know something but cannot fully express it. Strengthens one's relationship to one's inner voice, enabling a clear and unconfused expression of spirituality.

Lady's Mantle – For those who are scattered or confused. Develops sensitivity or self awareness. Imparts a feeling of strength and protection.

Lobelia – For confusion or uncertainty about one's feelings, ideas or opinions; for lack of clarity about goals. Stimulates courage to express, own, and speak the truth regarding one's self.

White Columbine – For those who feel uncertain or confused in life choices; for extreme ambivalence over a choice between two careers or life-changing options. Provides insight into one's true identity and highest purpose.

CONNECTION – SEE "RELATIONSHIPS"

CONTROL

Black Cohosh – For fear of being controlled by strong personalities; for those caught in controlling, abusive relationships. Treats the underlying fears, balancing one to be able to include a healthier range of responses to strong personalities.

Blessed Thistle – For fear of life and forces beyond one's control. Eases these fears, helping one to be more able to flow with life, accepting the possibility of earthly happiness.

Bull Thistle –For fears of being controlled by others. Strengthens anchoring forces and releases fears.

Golden Amaranthus – For those who over-control. Develops awareness of the power of the higher self. Develops ways to flow with the currents and tune into the ease of life.

Lilac – For those who over-rely on their own resources and have difficulty in asking for help, or even accepting help that is offered. Develops a healthy balance between self-reliance and reliance on others.

Milk Thistle – For those who feel they are taken advantage of, which gives rise to anger or resentment.

Motherwort– For those who feel controlled by others or attract controlling and abusive personalities. Helps one learn constructive, assertive behavior to set healthy, appropriate boundaries.

Solomon's Seal – For adapting to fluctuations, surprises, and changes that cannot be foreseen or controlled.

COMMUNITY EXPERIENCE – SEE "GROUP EXPERIENCE"

COUNSELING – SEE "THERAPY"

COURAGE

Black Currant – Gives the soul courage to go beyond internal fears and conflicts related to fears of abandonment or non-existence.

Borage – For the discouraged, burdened, depressed, melancholic, or fatalistic. Gives peace, lightness, and courage.

Lovage – For fear of risk or taking action; for low confidence, feelings of lack of safety. Helps one move into the world with a sense of safety, joy, and confidence.

Sumac – For discouragement, hopelessness, loss of motivation, resignation; for feeling like giving up. Strengthens one's ability to hold onto one's drive and sustain energy.

CREATIVITY – SEE "INSPIRATION"

CYNICISM (SEE ALSO "PESSIMISM," "TRUST")

Bluebell – For those who dwell in the negative and cannot cycle out of cynicism. Offers access to more positive aspects of one's personality.

Elecampagne – For those who are cynical, unable to accept compliments, or who identify with negative aspects of their personality. Helps one transition into a new identity, leaving older, negative imprints behind.

Fraxinella – For general cynicism about life; for those who hold grudges, feel stuck and unable to cope with life. Energies of frustration are dislodged and can be moved out of the energy field.

Indian Tobacco – For those who are overly cynical about spirituality. Relieves fears around spiritual experiences or ideas, often bringing to the conscious mind information related to their origin.

Jack-in-the-pulpit – For the spiritually jaded and cynical. Strengthens one's relationship to one's inner voice, enabling the expression of personal and authentic spirituality.

Marshmallow – For those who are cynical or closed to emotions. Softens one's mental body and interactions with people.

Star Jasmine – For cynicism and fatalism. Uplifts and spiritualizes one's perspective.

White Columbine – For cynicism related to self-doubt and feeling "lost." Provides a reassurance that "all is well" and unfolding in life. A quiet strength and acceptance develops.

Wood Betony – For cynicism about ability of oneself and others to change. Stimulates higher reasoning, allowing it to guide one in situations. The lower nature has less control and more ability to evolve.

DEATH AND DYING (SEE ALSO "GRIEF")

Black Currant – For fears of death and of not existing; for profound questions about life and death. Gives courage to go beyond internal fears and conflicts, and so to continue one's journey into truth, light and meaning. Eases the fears and overwhelming dread of those who are dying and do not believe in the survival of the soul after death.

Blessed Thistle – Helps ease the fear of life, as well as the fear of death. Useful for hospice workers; helps the individual who is passing to feel a closer connection to God. Helps family members feel more the mystery and love than the fear and sadness associated with this process.

Golden Amaranthus – Eases transitions through remembrance of the power of the soul in survival over physical death; for learning to let go of over-control; becoming aware of the power of the higher self, and that we are protected and guided on the highest level.

Indian Pipe – For those who can't feel the presence of Love or God; who feel unloved or lonely. Develops a sensitivity and receptivity to the presence of universal love in every moment.

Indian Tobacco – For fear of death. Helps to steady irrational fears or confusions. Helps to relieve buried fears regarding one's relationship to God, to spirituality, or to the world beyond the physical.

Onion – For all stages of the grieving process, as well as for unresolved grief, unexpressed sadness, or the reluctance or inability to cry. Helps one access the emotion that is present, then express it deeply and completely, and then move the grief-emotion out of the system.

DECISION-MAKING – SEE "MANIFESTATION"

DEPENDENCE / INDEPENDENCE

Bull Thistle – For those who feel controlled, or confined by loss of independence. Releases negative past experiences with structure or authority.

Butterfly Weed – For people who have difficulty giving up independence in relationships. Eases fear of being hurt or trapped and allows for more maturity and deeper relationship.

Golden Amaranthus – For those who tend to "do it all" themselves, as they are often disappointed in or mistrustful of others; for those who have a strong belief in and success through their own abilities and resources. Aids one in letting go of over-control, and constant vigilance. Helps one trust, enjoy, "let go and let God."

Lady's Mantle – For the overly dependent. Imparts a feeling of strength and protection, which supports one's ability to contain and to develop feminine strength.

Lilac – For the overly independent individual who is unable to allow help from others as well as for the overly-reliant individual. Assists in developing qualities of true balanced self-reliance and reliance on others.

Motherwort – For those who are overly dependent on what another person wants; for those who feel threatened and can't say no. Balances inner softness with strength. Helps with assertiveness and setting healthy boundaries.

Water Lily – For needy personalities who are dependent on attention from others. Offers a sense of self-sufficiency and fulfillment.

White Columbine – For those who don't trust themselves and are overly dependent on feedback from others. Provides a reassurance that "all is well" and unfolding in life.

DEPRESSION

Borage – For depression, sadness, loss of hope; for those who feel tired of their life. Offers a feeling of presence, groundedness, embodiment, even stoutheartedness. Stimulates courage to face challenges.

Bluebell – For those who dwell in the negative and cannot cycle out of cynicism; for grumpiness, withdrawal or aloofness. Provides access to more positive aspects of the personality.

Fraxinella – For depression surrounding trauma, feeling unable to cope with life or to change patterns and behaviors. Helps release stuck, heavy, or buried energies, offering a feeling of deep relief.

Golden Amaranthus – For depression along with worries about what might happen, for intense swings of energy and depletion, for those who are unable to rest because they are always "on guard" and rely only on themselves. Helps one trust, enjoy, relax, and go with the flow.

Habanero Pepper – For depression, along with the inability to feel joy or enthusiasm; for sluggishness or escapist tendencies. Catalyses movement of repressed energies related to trauma to the surface, creating more room for the circulation of soul energies and relieving depression.

Horseradish – For depression along with feelings of lethargy, stagnation, power-lessness, lack of vigor, obsessive thinking patterns; inability to change or have the life one wants. Confidence and vigor improve.

Indian Pipe – For those who feel unloved, lonely, or that they need more love; for those who feel depressed by many conditions in the world. Develops an awareness and receptivity to the presence of universal love which heals or eases many afflictions related to grief, loss, loneliness, or alienation.

Lemon Balm – For the anxiety that accompanies depression. Calms the mind.

Pink Lady's Slipper – For depression associated with trouble fitting in or expressing one's inner awareness; for alienation, obsessive, or suicidal thoughts.

Star Jasmine – For depression from feeling overburdened or constant frustration. Helps lighten feelings of somberness, heaviness, or fatigue. Brings the joy of spirit closer to the physical.

DISAPPOINTMENT – SEE "DISCOURAGEMENT"

DISCOURAGEMENT / DISAPPOINTMENT

Borage – For discouragement related to boredom or repetition or doing what one does not like to do; for sadness, depression, hopelessness.

Butterfly Weed – For fear and sadness when initial stages of "being in love" shift; for those who are consistently discouraged by the ending of the "highs" or roman-tic stages of relationships.

Golden Amaranthus – For continual disappointment with others who do not perform in a way that meets one's standards; for feelings as if the forces of fate or evil are conspiring against personal success.

Indian Pipe – For those who feel frustrated and disappointed by relationships; for those who can't understand or accept baser human emotions and actions, and feel saddened and depressed by many conditions in the world.

Onion – For children during disappointment or loss. Releases sadness. Supports inner-child work.

Sumac – For feelings of discouragement that accompany working on a task or project for a long time.

DREAMS – SEE "SLEEP"

EASE OF LIFE

Blessed Thistle – For fears of fate and power. Renews one's ability to flow with life. Helps one recognize that the powers that control our lives are wise and loving in nature.

Blue Vervain – For those who feel obliged to live their lives as leaders, role mod-els, or providers; for those who cannot yield to a safer, healthier, more practical approach because of pride, ambition or role identity; for those who always feel that "the buck stops with them."

Fraxinella – For those who feel frustrated, unable to cope with life. Offers relief from frustration. Heavy and stuck energies are released, allowing new ideas and possibilities to emerge.

Golden Amaranthus – For those who feel a deep internal struggle with life and a general sense of aloneness. Reawakens the awareness that one is guided and protected. Enables one to relax and tune into the ease of life.

Habanero Pepper – For those unable to feel joy or enthusiasm; for lethargy, sluggishness. Catalyzes movement of repressed energies related to trauma to the surface, creating more room for the circulation of soul energies.

Horseradish – Old recurring thoughts or ideas receive energy, encouraging action or release. One feels more power/energy to act.

Lemon Balm – Produces a calm that allows deeper exploration or work; one's mind remains keen while enveloped by peacefulness; useful in combination with remedies that catalyze movement or stir emotion.

Lovage – For moving into the world with a sense of safety and joy. Develops a sense of exhilaration and confidence in walking one's path and in taking action.

Missouri Primrose – For those who overwork and postpone enjoyment. Develops ones ability to self-nurture and enjoy life.

Pink Amaranthus – For developing ease in relationships.

Star Jasmine –For feelings of somberness, heaviness or fatigue; for depression from feeling overburdened. Helps lighten one's mood, and brings the joy of spirit closer to the physical.

Water Lily – For those who attract drama; for those who rely on acting out extreme emotional states in order to control situations. Offers emotional ease.

Wood Betony – For those who struggle to change or control behavior. Struggle with oneself is eased as higher reasoning is stimulated to guide the individual. The lower nature has less control over a situation.

ELDERS – SEE "AGING"

ENTHUSIASM –SEE "ENERGY," "JOY"

EMPATHY

Celandine – Enhances communication, understanding and empathy.

Hemp Agrimony – For those who are unable to feel closeness to others; those who feel alienated. Helps one access and develop the ability to connect to others.

Skullcap – Increases awareness of one's intuitive response to others. Helps one to feel and know another from the other's perspective. Enhances empathy in the healing process.

ENGAGEMENT WITH LIFE – SEE ALSO "FEAR," "GROUNDING," "RELATIONSHIP," "RESISTANCE"

Black Cohosh – For those who avoid confrontation. Provides clarity, lifting the spell and showing people and situations for what they are and not what they pretend to be. Helps one to remain engaged in dialogue, conflict, or negotiation without a reflex to avoid or disengage.

Black Currant – For inability to focus on daily matters, which had previously held the individual's interest, when ideas of self and reality are challenged.

Fraxinella – For those who avoid dealing with recent trauma. Eases trauma and keeps the energies of hurt and pain from sinking into the subconscious.

Habanero Pepper – For escapist tendencies. Provides stability and balance to "wandering souls."

Horseradish – For those who avoid confronting problems due to feeling powerless. Feelings of frustration and powerlessness are eased and a person is likely to feel more confidence.

Milk Thistle – For those who avoid feeling or dealing with anger. Releases and transforms lower emotions such as displaced or unconscious anger into loving energies.

Onion – For those who avoid dealing with sadness. Helps to access the emotion, express it deeply and completely, and move the grief-emotion out of the system.

Stinging Nettle – For those who suppress fear, anger, and sadness from loss of family unit in childhood.

Skullcap – For retreat, resignation or numbness to others and life events. Allows the soul's natural sensitivities to the self and to others to open.

ENERGY (SEE ALSO "EXHAUSTION")

Golden Amaranthus – For those who are tired, have difficulty resting and/or have intense swings of energy and depletion because they are always "on guard" and rely only on themselves. Reawakens the awareness that we are guided and protected, enabling one to relax and move with the flow of life. In this vibration, vitality and a relaxed energy flourish.

Habanero Pepper – For lethargy, sluggishness, difficulty concentrating or remembering, Catalyzes movement of repressed energies related to trauma to the surface, creating more room for the circulation of soul energies.

Horseradish – For those who feel stuck or lethargic. Old recurring thoughts or ideas receive energy to surface for action or release. One feels more power/energy to act.

Lemon Balm – For inability to relax; for fears related to resting. Provides a natural and deep relaxation, by easing the velocity of the mind, which can be agitated by fears that reside in the subconscious.

Lovage – For harnessing thought energy into action. Develops a sense of safety, exhilaration, and joy as one moves in the world, and confidence in taking action.

Lungwort – For moving energy blockages, and the symptoms they can intensify. Helps energy flow properly in rhythm with the breath. Adds strength and stamina to the entire physical system.

Star Jasmine – For feelings of heaviness or fatigue. Helps lighten one's mood. Brings the joy of spirit closer to the physical.

Sumac – For discouragement, disillusionment, or the wish to give up. Strengthens one's ability to sustain drive and energy. Helps one continue to strive or work towards a goal.

Teasel – For emotional pain that causes energy depletion. Helps hold and maintain energy within the system.

ENJOYMENT SEE "EASE OF LIFE"

ESCAPISM – SEE "ENGAGEMENT WITH LIFE," "RESISTANCE"

EXHAUSTION

Blue Vervain – For those who work until exhausted. For those who push the body to the limit. Helps one develop a more self-nurturing lifestyle.

Golden Amaranthus – For swings of intense energy and depletion; for inability to rest. Helps one learn to maintain energy through a rhythm of ease.

Lovage – For those who feel heavy or lethargic. Develops a sense of exhilaration as well as safety in taking action.

Star Jasmine – For feelings of somberness, heaviness or fatigue; depression from feeling overburdened. Lightens one's mood and brings the joy of spirit closer to the physical.

Sumac – For those who are exhausted and disheartened; for those who feel that they have somehow missed life or have been passed by. Brings a strength and stamina to the system.

Teasel – For emotional exhaustion; for trying too hard in a task, causing energy depletion. Helps one learn to use energy in a balanced and judicious manner.

EXHILARATION – SEE "JOY"

EXPLOITATION – SEE "PROTECTION"

EXPRESSION – SEE "COMMUNICATION" AND "SELF-EXPRESSION"

FAITH – SEE "SPIRITUALITY," "TRUST"

FAMILY (SEE ALSO CHILDREN, ADOLESCENCE)

Canada Thistle – Letting go of pain, guilt or trauma which has been group or family inflicted.

Japanese Knotweed – Useful for when there is family disharmony. Enhances sympathetic awareness. Also for when an adult joins a family as a partner to another adult with children. Many stresses are relieved and adaptation time is shortened greatly. Best results occur when all family members are able to take the essence.

Hyssop – For those who were brought up in guilt-based families, when there is an awareness that what has been taught was harmful, but there is still a strong reflex towards guilt. Releases imprints of guilt. Reawakens impulses of worthiness and receiving. One's orientation changes from blame to acceptance.

Lady's Mantle – For those who fear leaving home. Imparts a feeling of strength and protection that supports one's ability to contain and to use feminine energies.

Milk Thistle – For those who learned unhealthy ways of dealing with anger in their family of origin.

Motherwort – For unhealthy boundary issues learned in one's family of origin.

Skullcap – For women who have given up children for adoption or who have had abortions.

Stinging Nettle – For releasing family traumas related to abandonment or family breakup.

FATALISM – SEE "PESSIMISM"

FATIGUE – SEE "EXHAUSTION"

FEAR (SEE ALSO "COURAGE")

Black Cohosh – For fears of violence, strong personalities, or being hurt. Eases timidity and fear of confrontations.

Black Currant – For fears of abandonment or death; fears of risk, ending relationships, crowds, or competition; for unexplained fears and fears of change in general.

Blessed Thistle – For fears of life, fate, dying, heights, power or law enforcement; agoraphobia, fear of moving with life. Eases guilt and fear of punishment. Eases fear of forces beyond one's control.

Borage – Offers groundedness, embodiment, steadfast courage, and stoutheartedness when facing fears.

Bull Thistle – For fears of being trapped in places or situations. Releases fears of authorities and being controlled by others.

Butterfly Weed – For fear of commitment in relationships.

Celandine – For fear of speaking or of being misunderstood.

Elecampagne – For fear of losing control; fears of driving or being in open spaces; fears of driving over bridges.

Golden Amaranthus – For worries about what might happen, fear of fate, and sometimes spirituality; for fear of failure.

Gravel Root – For various types of fears related to aloneness and being alone.

Hemp Agrimony – For many social fears; for those who have a fear or feeling that tells them it is unsafe to be with others.

Hyssop – For fear of punishment, pleasure, or success, for feelings of foreboding, or fears that something must go wrong.

Indian Tobacco – For irrational fears or confusions; for releasing subconscious fears of spirituality.

Lemon Balm – For fears related to resting. Eases mental turbulence.

Scarlet Pimpernel – Helps relieve fears resulting from suppressing emotions.

FLEXIBILITY (SEE ALSO BOUNDARIES)

Golden Amaranthus – For willfulness; over-reliance on one's self; frustration with others, time, and events. Helps one move with the flow of life, and let go of over-control.

Lilac – For rigidity, resists changing plans or standards, is easily frustrated.

Marshmallow – Teaches how to soften interactions with those who we do not feel connected to. Helps one to feel ease around people, and especially those that we do not like.

Solomon's Seal – For inflexible people who cannot deal with change or things going wrong. Helps one adapt to fluctuations, surprises and changes that can not be foreseen or controlled.

FEMININE ENERGIES

Blackberry Lily – For treating feminine energies damaged by sexual abuse.

Lady's Mantle – For those who have an imbalance in masculine and feminine energies. Strengthens one's ability to contain and to use feminine energy.

Marshmallow – For accessing softer energies.

Motherwort – For balancing inner softness with strength.

Skullcap – Aids recovery for women who have given up children for adoption or who have had abortions.

FOCUS – SEE "CLARITY," "CONCENTRATION," "STUDY"

FORGIVENESS – SEE "ANGER," "PEACEMAKING"

FRIENDSHIP – SEE "RELATIONSHIPS"

FRUSTRATION

Celandine – For frustrations around communication, either difficulty getting a point across or in receivinng messages. Enhances sensitivity to reception and transmission of information.

Fraxinella – For feeling frustrated; for frustrations that conspire to lock a person into a belief that no relief or change is possible.

Golden Amaranthus – For those easily or regularly frustrated or worried about what might happen; frustration is with time and events. Helps one move with the flow of life and let go of over-control. The stress of attachment to daily performance and success is eased considerably. One can experience setbacks or even failure without obsessive frustrations.

Indian Pipe – For those who feel frustrated and disappointed by relationships; can't understand or accept baser human emotions and actions, for those heart-oriented beings who have tremendous difficulty relating to the absence of love and warmth in their environment.

Lilac – For those who become frustrated because of too much to do; for those who cannot rely on others.

Lovage – For those who feel frustrated, disconnected or unhappy about their situation, or for those who feel their life is going nowhere.

Onion – For the early stages of grief when one can feel frustration and anger. Helps the entire grieving process: accessing one's emotions, expressing them and moving the grief-emotions out of the system.

Marshmallow – For those who are frustrated and "hard" in their interactions. Helps one soften interactions and feel at ease around people one does not feel connected to nor like.

Milk Thistle – For those who over-react when frustrated; for repressed anger.

Jack-in-the-pulpit – For those who are frustrated by religious thought. Strengthens the relationship to one's inner voice, making the expression of authentic spirituality more possible. Helps one resolve conflicts between past spiritual experiences and present spiritual insight.

Solomon's Seal – For those who frustrate easily. Helps one adapt to fluctuations, surprises and changes that can not be foreseen or controlled.

Wood Betony – For frustrated idealism, for frustrations related to feeling stuck and unable to change.

GRIEF (SEE ALSO "DEATH AND DYING")

Borage – For relief from the heaviness of grief. Offers a groundedness and courage that helps one stay engaged with life and have hope.

Golden Amaranthus – Eases transitions through remembrance of the power of the soul to survive physical death.

Gravel Root – For general loneliness or a lingering pain of loss of a spouse or close companion.

Hyssop – For guilt feelings around the loss of a loved one. Releases guilt and shame.

Indian Pipe – For stages when one feels unloved, or needs more love. Eases many afflictions related to grief, loss, separation, or loneliness.

Marshmallow – For those who harden as a way of protecting themselves from harm or grief; for those who can't feel emotions. Softens the emotional body, allowing one to feel grief and sadness.

Onion – For all stages of the grieving process; for unresolved grief, unexpressed sadness, or inability to cry.

Stinging Nettle – For releasing pain and grief related to partings and endings; for healing deep hurt from abandonment or childhood tragedy.

Star Jasmine – Helps one feel the deeper or spiritual meaning behind painful events.

Sumac – For endurance during long grieving processes.

Teasel – For grief that is recent, intense, and drains energy suddenly and dramatically. Helps to restore and rebalance energy loss.

GROUNDING

Borage – For the discouraged and heavy-hearted. Gives a feeling of groundedness, and embodiment, helping the conscious mind to have hope.

Bull Thistle – For fears of being trapped or controlled by others. Strengthens anchoring forces and releases fears.

Habanero Pepper – For separation, drifting during strong emotions. Holds one in connection to the physical. Promotes clarity and presence, at the same time stimulates movement of repressed feelings.

Indian Tobacco – For keeping balance in the mental body during expanded states. Helps to steady irrational fears or confusions.

Lemon Balm – For strong and intense emotions. One's mind remains keen while enveloped by calmness and peacefulness.

Potato – For grounding as one expands, awakens, and develops; also for the tendency to sublimate or romanticize painful experiences. Brings a sense of stability in the growth process by providing a deep reference point of self when new experiences pull one off center.

GRUDGES – SEE "OBSESSIONS"

GROUP / COMMUNITY EXPERIENCE

Canada Thistle – For letting go of pain, guilt, or trauma that has been group inflicted.

Celandine – For any breakdown in communication between individuals or factions within a larger group. Enhances sensitivity to feelings, intentions, and orientations of others. Useful in negotiation,.

Elecampagne – For those who feel odd or different from others; uncomfortable in group situations. Offers a comfort with one's own unique identity, aiding social turmoil and ability to connect with others.

Fraxinella – For working groups to assist in moving past or resolving issues. Helps people to redirect their energies. Releases and replaces frustration with more positive feelings towards success.

Gravel Root – For those who fear being alone but do not feel safe in groups.

Hemp Agrimony – For those who lose themselves in groups or do not feel connected to others.

Jack-in-the-pulpit – For those who are estranged from organized spiritual or religious groups or feel animosity towards spiritual leaders. Strengthens one's expression of a personal and authentic spirituality. Organized groups and religions receive the benefit of "inspired" expression, and the individual feels accepted and expressed.

Japanese Knotweed – For building agreement and harmony in groups. Also for when new members join a well-established group or when there is a change in membership of any kind. Enhances group experiences.

Lobelia – For those who keep silent in groups; for those who do not internally align with the conscious values of a group and "go underground" with their truths. Offers courage to express, own, and speak the truth regarding one's self.

Pink Lady's Slipper – For gifted people who have trouble fitting in or expressing the awareness they hold within. Helps one to realize the beauty and power of one's own being. This in turn helps one to be more expressive in groups. Acts as a longer term evolutionary therapy.

Skullcap – Increases awareness of one's intuitive response to others. Enhances group empathy.

GUILT

Blessed Thistle – For guilt and fear of punishment. Enhances feelings of enjoying life; eases fear of forces beyond one's control.

Canada Thistle – For letting go of pain, guilt or trauma that has been group or family inflicted.

Hyssop – For those who have built personalities and lifestyles around guilt imprints. Cleanses and releases imprints of guilt, shame, and unworthiness. Reawakens impulses of worthiness and receiving.

Missouri Primrose – For guilt indoctrination, low self-esteem, inability to receive complements. Helps one accept and receive love, friendship, goodness, pleasure, and other forms of self-nurturing.

HABIT PATTERNS

Fraxinella – For feeling unable to get past or resolve an issue or habit. Releases frustration, often offering insight, new ideas, and possibilities that have not previously been considered.

Hyssop – For self-sabotage; for habit patterns stemming from guilt-based families, philosophies or religions.

Horseradish – For obsessive thinking patterns. Old recurring thoughts or ideas come forward for action or release.

Milk Thistle – For those who have habits of repressing anger, then losing control.

Scarlet Pimpernel – For many aspects of difficult emotions, such as obsession, anxiety, and fear. Helps one understand and transform intense emotions.

Wood Betony – For those who feel trapped by desires, unable to change or control behavior. Stimulates the higher reasoning to guide the individual in a situation, giving the lower nature less control over a situation.

Wormwood – For those who feel stuck in old habits or in the past. Breaks and releases old patterns or unconscious imprints.

HEALING ARTS /HEALERS /HEALING (SEE ALSO "THERAPY," "PROTECTION")

Celandine – For therapists and healers of all types. Enhances sensitivity to reception and transmission of information.

Potato – For use after any deep healing experience. Gently brings one back into the body, into one's "normal reality," where one can reflect about and integrate the experience.

Skullcap – For difficulties in feeling empathy or connecting. Helps therapists form relationships with clients.

Star Jasmine – For healers of all kinds who may occasionally feel depressed, overwhelmed, or even fatalistic from having such close and regular association with these energies.

Sumac – For maintaining connection with the heart during difficult transitions in recovery. For healers who struggle internally with the difficulty of their work.

HEARTEDNESS – HEART CONNECTION

Butterfly Weed – Strengthens the ability of the heart to hold the love vibration.

Hemp Agrimony – For those feel disconnected and alienated. Develops heart connection with others.

Indian Pipe – For stages when stress, cold efficiency, intolerance, and conflict overshadow love, patience, and harmony. One develops a sensitivity and receptivity to feeling the presence of universal love.

Lungwort – Helps release blocked emotions that may be the cause of heart problems.

Marshmallow – For the hard-hearted. Strengthens one's ability to receive impulses from the heart and choose higher emotional values. Softens the entire emotional system.

Milk Thistle – For angry personality types who develop heart problems.

Pink Amaranthus – For those who are afraid to open the heart for fear of vulnerability, weakness or hurt. Strengthens, nurtures and heals the ability to trust love as an active force in one's life.

Scarlet Pimpernel – Helps with many aspects of difficult emotions such as obsession, anxiety and fear. Releases blocked energy in the heart. Helps one understand and transform intense emotions.

Skullcap – For difficulties in feeling empathy or connecting. Helps one form heart-connections to others.

Sumac – For maintaining connection with the heart during difficult phases. Helps one realize that what is held in the heart is important and to use it as energy to continue striving towards a goal.

HOPE

Borage – For discouragement and loss of hope. Offers a feeling of presence, groundedness, embodiment, even stoutheartedness. Stimulates courage to face challenges and to have hope.

Indian Pipe – For stages when stress, cold efficiency, intolerance, and conflict can overshadow love, patience, and harmony; for those who feel saddened and depressed by many conditions in the world.

Pink Amaranthus – Heals hopelessness that results from failed relationships.

Star Jasmine – For those who are looking for more inspiration in their problem solving processes. Adds clarity to intellectual pursuits and increases insight and illumination to areas where the intellect receives inspiration from the intuition.

Sumac – For those who feel like giving up. Maintains hope and endurance during long trials.

Wormwood – Helps release hopelessness.

IDENTITY

Black Currant – For deep fears related to identity shifts and crises; for the fear of non-existence or losing the ego. Opens one to soul identity.

Elecampagne – For times when new feelings, talents, insights are awakened. Helps one to identify more deeply with newly discovered aspects of one's self.

Jack-in-the-pulpit – For developing one's authentic and spiritual identity. Strengthens one's relationship to one's inner voice, making the expression of an authentic spirituality more possible.

Pink Lady's Slipper – For identity crises; for those who don't fit in. One's true identity on the earth plane is accessed.

Missouri Primrose – For those who identify with negative self-concepts. Develops one's identity of self-worth.

Skullcap – For those whose essential self has retreated from consciousness. One's feelings, interests, preferences, and self-nurturing abilities are regained, as well as an increased empathy for others.

White Columbine – For those who feel uncertain or lost in life choices. Provides insight into true identity and highest purpose.

Wormwood – For lingering or negative identities based on past mistreatment. Moves out old patterns. Releases unconscious imprints.

INCARNATION

Blackberry Lily – For past life work when some event from another lifetime appears to be interfering with relationships in the present incarnation.

Borage – Offers a feeling of presence, groundedness, embodiment, stouthearted-ness to assist the conscious mind in choosing to stay incarnated and to have hope.

Comfrey – Assists conscious energy in penetrating deeper into the subconscious.

Habanero Pepper – Releases trauma blocking proper incarnation.

Indian Tobacco – For unexplained fears that seem to stem from memories from other lifetimes. Relieves fears around spiritual experiences or ideas, often bringing to the conscious mind information related to its origin.

Lovage – One receives a greater commitment to one's incarnation through the joy of success.

Lungwort – Helps one who blocks energy, allowing deeper incarnation.

Marshmallow – Softens the emotional body allowing deeper incarnation.

Pink Lady's Slipper – Helps special or higher vibrating souls to incarnate.

Potato – Helps one return to incarnation after a deep spiritual experience.

Solomon's Seal – Helps one to accept incarnation by accepting failure and imperfection.

White Columbine – Deeper commitment to incarnation comes from realizing one's life path.

INNER VOICE – SEE "IDENTITY," "SELF-EXPRESSION"

INSPIRATION

Celandine – For self-expression. Enhances many aspects of communication by receiving inspiration or higher thoughts. Enhances the work of musicians, actors, artists and writers.

Elecampagne – For times when new feelings, talents, insights are awakened. Helps one identify more deeply with newly discovered power and beauty in one's self.

Indian Pipe – For stages when stress, cold efficiency, and conflict overshadow love, patience, and harmony. Expands awareness of the presence of universal love, and the opportunity to use this energy.

Jack-in-the-Pulpit – For those unsure how to integrate spiritual inspiration with day-to-day expression. Strengthens one's relationship to the inner voice, enabling the inspired expression of authentic spirituality.

Lady's Mantle – For blocked creativity, lack of confidence; for those who feel unexpressed. Supports the expression of the feminine energies, such as empathy, creativity, intuition, wisdom, spirituality, for both men and women.

Lemon Balm – For those who feel blocked, with no inspiration. Enhances the creative process. Helps move tension and anxiety out so thatother levels of the mind can become active and express themselves.

Lobelia – For those who feel unable to express or hide their awareness. Inspires one to express the truth.

Pink Lady's Slipper –For artistic or gifted people who have trouble fitting in or expressing their awareness. Inspiration is made more available to the conscious mind for expression.

Star Jasmine – For those who feel blocked and are seeking inspiration in problem-solving. Adds clarity to intellectual pursuits and increases insight and illumination to areas where the intellect receives inspiration from the intuition.

Sumac – For those who feel like giving up. Inspires one to continue when faltering.

Wood Betony – For those who feel uninspired or stuck. Helps one wishing to solve a problem or issue have access to clear thinking and awareness. Works especially with artists, scientists, inventors, writers and philosophers. Enhances more inspired thinking.

INSIGHT – SEE "AWARENESS," "INSPIRATION"

INTOLERANCE – SEE "PREJUDICE"

INTUITION

Golden Amaranthus – For developing intuition regarding the "right" thing to do.

Indian Tobacco – For releasing fears related to the power of intuition.

Japanese Knotweed – For developing intuition in groups.

Skullcap – For strengthening one's intuitive response to others. Helps one to feel and know another from the other's perspective. Enhances empathy in the healing process.

Star Jasmine – For those seeking inspiration in problem solving. Adds clarity to intellectual pursuits and increases insight and intuition.

JEALOUSY

Lady's Mantle – For those who are envious of others. Imparts a feeling of strength and protection which supports the ability to contain and to use one's own feminine power.

Milk Thistle – For repressed anger, rage, and jealousy.

White Columbine – For jealousy and uncertainty. Provides a reassurance that "all is well" and unfolding in life. Feelings of inferiority and insecurity, yield to a quiet strength and acceptance.

JOY

Borage – For the discouraged, downcast, and joyless. Imparts happiness and contentment.

Lovage – For those unable to enjoy work or one's path in life. Develops a sense of safety, joy, and exhilaration as one moves into the world.

Indian Pipe – For stages when stress, cold efficiency, intolerance and conflict overshadow love, patience and harmony. Expands awareness of the presence of universal love, and with that joy.

Star Jasmine – For feelings of somberness, heaviness or fatigue and depression from feeling overburdened. Helps lighten emotions and brings the joy of spirit closer to the physical.

JUDGMENTAL – SEE "PREJUDICE," "TRUST"

LEADERSHIP (SEE ALSO "AUTHORITY," "AMBITION")

Blue Vervain – For those who misjudge themselves to be over-responsible and work too hard.

Celandine – Enhances communications. Assists individuals and couples to work through judgmental patterns.

Golden Amaranthus – For those who misjudge the presence of the divine assistance, working instead against the "flow" of life.

Jack-in-the-Pulpit – For those who are overly judgmental towards religions due to their own unexpressed spirituality.

Marshmallow – For those in authority who harden against the feeling of responsibility; for those in that are intolerant, narrow-minded, inflexible. Strengthens one's ability to receive impulses from the heart and choose higher emotional values.

LEARNING – SEE "STUDY," "AWARENESS"

LETHARGY – SEE "STAGNATION"

LINGERING EMOTIONS – SEE "RELEASE"

LONELINESS / ALONENESS

Black Currant – For those who fear of abandonment; feel invisible; feel slighted or ignored easily.

Elecampagne – For those who feel odd or different from others, uncomfortable in social situations. Aids in the ability to connect with others.

Golden Amaranthus – For a general sense of separateness and regular frustration; for those who over-rely on their own selves, are mistrustful and suspicious of others. Helps develop trust in others.

Gravel Root – For loneliness or fears related to aloneness; for anxiety about relationships. Eases fears and enhances one's ability to form solid, healthy, conscious connections with others, as well as to find solace in being alone.

Hemp Agrimony – For many social fears; for those who are shy or fearful of social contact; feeling disconnected, alienated or in exile. Eases feelings and perceptions of aloneness, or disconnectedness.

Indian Pipe – For those who feel lonely or unloved, frustrated and disappointed by relationships. Expands awareness of the love in every moment. Feeling the presence of love can heal or ease many afflictions related to grief, loss, separation, loneliness, or alienation.

Skullcap – For those who feel or need to be alone; for social anxieties. Allows the soul's natural sensitivities to the self and to others to open.

Water Lily – For those who crave attention from others. Offers a sense of self-sufficiency and fulfillment.

White Columbine – For those who feel lonely or confused about the direction of their life. For those searching for the right relationship. Offers insight to one's true identity and purpose and that "all is well" and unfolding in life.

Wood Betony – For those who prefer to be alone, but are working on authentic ways to connect with others. Clarifies the deeper meaning of relationships.

LOSS – SEE "GRIEF"

LOVE (SEE ALSO "ROMANTIC LOVE")

Hemp Agrimony – For many social fears. Opens one to a particular spectrum of the love vibration where one begins to understand the interconnectedness of all things through the heart. Previously undeveloped qualities of compassion, altruism, and leadership may emerge.

Indian Pipe – For those who feel lonely and that they need more love. For those who have tremendous difficulty relating to the absence of love and warmth in their environment. Also for those who are working to develop the vibration of unconditional love in their own being.

Marshmallow – For those who harden emotionally to protect themselves. Helps one feel impulses from the heart and to feel love even when one is hurt.

Milk Thistle – For deep anger, resentment or other held feelings that block the flow of love. Allows forgiveness to lead the way to a deeper experience of love. Provides a bridge to lessons of unconditional love.

Missouri Primrose – For those with low self esteem and difficulty in receiving love. Helps one to accept and receive love, friendship, pleasure and other forms of self-nurturing.

Pink Amaranthus – For those afraid to open the heart for fear of vulnerability, weakness, hurt. Balances tendencies to weaken, or give away strength in the process of giving love. Fosters a feeling of safety within the heart space.

Pink Lady's Slipper –For altruistic, spiritually-minded or gifted people who have trouble fitting in or expressing the love or joy they hold within.

Star Jasmine – For those seeking to uplift or add a spiritual perspective. Emotions become aligned with spirituality, love becomes unconditional.

MANIFESTATION

Elecampagne – For those who feel unable to change; for those who have difficulty identifying with success. Helps one transition into a new identity, leaving older, more negative imprints behind.

Fraxinella – For those who cannot get past or resolve an issue; for frustrations which create the belief that no relief or change is possible. Releases frustration, allowing flashes of insight, inspiration or creative solutions to emerge.

Horseradish – For those who feel powerless, stuck, or unable to have the life they want. Old recurring thoughts or ideas receive energy to come forward for action, release, or manifestation. Obsessive thinking patterns are discarded. Goal-directed energies are enhanced.

Lovage – For difficulty manifesting plans into action; for procrastination; for any stage of life exploration when one considers choices and the future. Helps create momentum for making change in a positive direction. Develops confidence in taking action.

Missouri Primrose – For self-sabotage, procrastination, postponing enjoyment. Helps one accept and receive love, friendship, goodness, pleasure, and other forms of self-nurturing. Vital energies taken in through self-nurturing are later converted into confidence and goal-directed activities.

Wood Betony – For those who struggle or feel unable to change. Stimulates higher reasoning, allowing it to act as a guide in situations. The lower nature has less control and is more ability to evolve.

MATERIALISM

Black Currant – For the over-rational; for those who tend towards extreme materialism, or secretly deny spiritual or metaphysical realities. Gives the courage and illumination needed to look at and integrate one's spiritual experience.

Blessed Thistle – For the very materialistic. Helps one open to possibilities of other levels of satisfaction.

Indian Tobacco – For those who are overly materialistic and avoid spirituality altogether. Helps to relieve fears or confusions around spiritual experiences or ideas.

Jack-in-the-pulpit – For the material-minded. Helps develop a more spiritual outlook through strengthening one's relationship to the inner voice.

Star Jasmine – For the agnostic, materialistic, narrow-minded. Uplifts or adds a spiritual perspective.

Stinging Nettle – For those who are stuck in materialistic viewpoints due to early childhood pain.

MEDITATION – SEE "SPIRITUALITY"

MID-LIFE CRISIS AND CONCERNS

Black Currant – For a mid-life crisis or any major change; for those who are disoriented or timid after an experience of growth or expansion. Gives one the courage to go beyond internal fears and conflicts to continue the journey into truth, light, and meaning.

Elecampagne – For mid-life or identity crises; for feeling misplaced.

Golden Amaranthus – For deep internal struggle, a sense of separateness, regular frustration; for those who are overworked, over-committed, unfocused or unexpressed. Eases transitions and struggles through the awareness that one is guided and protected. Helps one let down one's guard to enjoy, trust, and go with the flow.

Jack-in-the-pulpit – For the mid-life crisis, when one looks for deeper meanings in life. Strengthens one's inner "knowing." Helps one coordinate what one "feels" to be true with what one has "learned" is real.

Japanese Knotweed – For family issues during mid-life crises. Enhances sympathetic awareness.

Motherwort – For early menopause. Balances inner softness with strength. Imparts strength, assertiveness and ability to set healthy boundaries.

Pink Lady's Slipper – For mid-life crisis, and late-bloomers. Helps one realize the beauty and subtle power of one's being.

Sumac – For mid-life crises, when one is discouraged, disillusioned, or wants to give up. Also for any major life change when there is difficulty to look and plan ahead. Strengthens one's foundational rhythm in the ability to sustain drive and energy. Helps one to continue to strive or work towards any goal.

MISTRUST – SEE "TRUST," "CYNICISM"

MOTIVATION

Borage – Helps motivate those who are timid or fearful.

Lovage – For harnessing thought energy into action. Helps create momentum for making change in a positive direction. Develops confidence in taking action.

Golden Amaranthus – For the over use of will forces; for an over-reliance on oneself. Aids one in tuning into the ease of life and in developing ways to flow with the currents.

Horseradish – Helps motivate those who feel stuck or powerless.

Sumac – Helps motivate those who wish to give up.

NATURE AWARENESS & CONNECTION

Celandine – For those who feel frustrated or cut off from spiritual communication and communing with nature spirits; for those learning to connect as well as those practicing connection with nature spirits. Assists in adding clarity to intuitive information that one is receiving.

Hemp Agrimony – For those who feel disconnected alienated or in exile from the earth; for those who fear nature. Eases feelings and perceptions of aloneness, or disconnectedness.

Pink Lady's Slipper – Awakens the relationship with nature and acts as a focal point for the mysterious power of the forest. Offers the realization of the beauty of the earth and of human nature.

NEEDINESS

Lady's Mantle – For those who feel needy, indulge in private feelings of self-pity, or are overly dependent. Helps one feel more safe, secure, and stable. Strengthens the ability to contain and use feminine energies.

Pink Amaranthus – For those who are obsessive or aggressive in their search for a relationship. Helps one become aware of and utilize positive love energies rather than focusing on fears, doubts, and negativity.

Water Lily – For the needy personality; for those who crave attention, attract drama, or need to control and manipulate situations. Offers a sense of self-sufficiency, fulfillment, and emotional ease.

NEGATIVITY SEE "PESSIMISM"

OBSESSIONS

Blue Vervain – For those obsessed with work, responsibility, or success.

Fraxinella – For those who are obsessed with a past experience or hold grudges.

Golden Amaranthus – For obsessed perfectionists. Eases stress of attachment to daily performance and success. Helps one experience setbacks or even failure without obsessive frustrations.

Horseradish – For obsessive thinking patterns. For feeling powerless, stuck, or blaming others or fate for problems. Obsessive thinking patterns are discarded.

Hyssop – For perfectionism that is guilt-based. Helps "undo" some of the irrational footholds of judgment and self-condemnation, which in turn eases guilt and shame-based patterns.

Lilac – For those obsessed with the need to "do it all" themselves either due to very high standards, or low self-esteem. Helps one develop a healthy balance between self-reliance and reliance on others.

Marshmallow – For obsessions, inflexibility, holding grudges. Softens the entire emotional system so that emotions are released.

Scarlet Pimpernel – For obsession, anxiety and general displaced fear. Helps one understand and transform intense emotions.

Pink Amaranthus – For those who are obsessive or aggressive in their search for a relationship. Helps one become aware of and utilize positive love energies rather than focusing on fears, doubts, and negativity.

Pink Lady's Slipper – For obsessive thoughts associated with trouble fitting in or expressing one's inner awareness. Helps one recognize the beauty of one's being. Supports and strengthens the use of one's gentle and subtle power.

Teasel – For a long-standing obsessive thoughts that bring energy down. Helps to restore and rebalance energy loss.

Water Lily – For those obsessed with the need for attention, and who attract drama. Offers a sense of self-sufficiency, fulfillment, and emotional ease.

Wormwood – For lingering negative or unwanted thoughts, feelings, or habits. Clears out the psychic "debris" that remains in the energy field. Helpful when one has done some processing or therapeutic work.

OVERBURDENED – SEE "OVERWHELMED"

OVER-RATIONALISM – SEE "MATERIALISM"

OVERWHELMED / OVERBURDENED

Blue Vervain – For those who feel overwhelmed by a task, a responsibility, a job, or a project. Ease and versatility develop.

Golden Amaranthus – For the overworked and over-committed, for those who feel the need to "do it all themselves." Aids one in tuning into the ease of life and developing ways to flow with the currents.

Lemon Balm – For mental turbulence, anxiety, difficulty relaxing. Offers a calmness that provides protection against stress and breakdowns that one can experience when overloaded.

Star Jasmine – For feelings of heaviness or fatigue, depression from feeling over-burdened. Helps lighten feelings and brings the joy of spirit closer to the physical.

Teasel – For those who lose energy by trying too hard in a task or by over-giving in relationship. Helps one to learn to use energy in a balanced and judicious manner.

PAIN (EMOTIONAL)

Indian Pipe – For those who feel unloved, lonely, or need more love; for heart-oriented people who have tremendous difficulty relating to the absence of love and warmth in their environment. Develops a sensitivity and receptivity to the presence of universal love in every moment, which, in turn, can heal or ease many afflictions related to grief, loss, separation, loneliness, or alienation.

Marshmallow – For those who harden their emotions to protect against hurt and emotional pain; for emotionally repressed individuals, those who have difficulty in letting go of past hurts. Develops emotional resilience through the ability to feel intensely and then let go.

Onion – For all aspects of the grieving process; for unresolved or unexpressed grief or sadness. Helps one to first access and then express in order to release painful grief.

Scarlet Pimpernel – For many aspects of intense emotions, such as obsession, anxiety, and fear. Helps one understand and transform painful emotions. Releases blocked energy in the heart.

Stinging Nettle – For untreated childhood pain, when events trigger overly intense emotions; for any type of emotional pain experienced in the present. Eases pain and grief and aids in healing deep hurt from abandonment.

Teasel – For anger that is recent, intense, and drains energy suddenly and dramatically; for energy loss due to fighting and arguments. Helps to rebalance energy loss due to emotional pain.

PANIC

Black Current – For panic related to identity shifts and crises; for the fear of non-existence or losing the ego.

Blue Vervain – Treats panic; for fears associated with failure.

Borage – For courage in the face of panic.

Bull Thistle – For panic and fears of being trapped in places or situations; for claustrophobia. Strengthens anchoring forces, releases fears of being controlled by others.

Butterfly Weed – For fear and panic related to commitment; for fear of losing freedom.

Elecampagne – For fear of losing control, fear and panic related to bridges or highways.

Lemon Balm – Produces a calm that allows deeper emotional exploration; one's mind remains keen while enveloped by peacefulness.

PASSION –SEE "JOY," "INSPIRATION"

PEACE / PEACE-MAKING
Black Cohosh – For those who act in the role of peacekeeper. Enhances a healthy range of responses to strong personalities. Allows one to remain engaged in dialogue, conflict, or negotiation without a reflex to avoid or disengage.
Borage – Instills feelings of calm and peacefulness.
Golden Amaranthus – For those who fear fate, worry about what might happen, or are easily or regularly frustrated. Develops a feeling of peace, ease, and flowing with life.
Indian Pipe – For those who have tremendous difficulty relating to the absence of love in their environment, such as those saddened and depressed by many conditions in the world; for pacifists.
Japanese Knotweed – For group-related discord. Harmonizes group energy, producing a sympathetic bond among all members.
Lemon Balm – For strong and intense emotions. One's mind remains keen while enveloped by calmness and peacefulness.
Marshmallow – For those who refuse to listen or compromise; for those who harden their conscience against the feeling of responsibility when hearing about injustice in the world. Strengthens one's ability to choose higher emotional values. Teaches one to feel at ease with those one does not like.
Milk Thistle – Letting go of deep anger, resentment, or other held feelings that block the flow of love, allowing forgiveness to lead the way to a deeper experience of love.
Motherwort – For many phases of conflict resolution. Balances inner softness with strength. Imparts strength, assertiveness, and the ability to set healthy boundaries.
Sumac – For those who feel like giving up; that the meaning for continuing their struggle is gone. One feels strength and a peacefulness to continue.
Wood Betony – For frustrated idealism. Stimulates the higher functioning of the psyche, such as inspired thinking. The feeling of struggle diminishes and a sense of peace and certainty emerges.

PERFECTIONISM (SEE ALSO OBSESSIONS)
Lilac – For perfectionists and those who tend to "do it all" themselves, either due to very high standards or low self-esteem; for those who do not feel comfortable or worthy to receive assistance from others. Assists in developing qualities of true balanced self-reliance and reliance on others.
Golden Amaranthus – For perfectionists and those who are frustrated and disappointed that others do not perform in a way that meets their standards. Opens one to the awareness that we are guided and protected, helping one to relax and flow with the currents.
Pink Amaranthus – For those who have overly-high standards for a relationship, and so prevent relationships from developing. Helps one become aware of and utilize positive love energies rather than focusing on fears, doubts, and negativity.

Solomon's Seal – For those with high standards, who become frustrated when things do not go as planned. Produces a strength that comes from the flexibility.

PESSIMISM (SEE ALSO "CYNICISM")

Black Currant – For those who carry a general existential gloom, feel dread, expect failure, or are cynical. Eases the deep fear of non-existence. Gives one courage to go beyond this internal fear and conflict to continue the journey into truth, light, and the meaning of eternity.

Blessed Thistle – For those who feel that God or the Powers that guide all things are cruel or impersonal; trepidation of fate. Eases these fears, helping a person to be more able to flow with life, accepting the possibility of earthly happiness.

Golden Amaranthus – For those who fear fate, worry about what might happen, or are generally mistrustful and suspicious. Offers the awareness that one is guided and protected, easing fears and worries.

Star Jasmine – For fatalism, pessimism, narrow-mindedness. Uplifts and spiritualizes one's perspective.

PHYSICAL AILMENTS – ENERGETIC/ EMOTIONAL CONNECTIONS*

Essences for physical presentations are most effective when the personality characteristics described in the profiles accompany the physical symptoms. The essences are not represented here as a cure for symptoms themselves, but rather as a complementary therapy, which can ease the energetic problems that are a source of the physical disease.

Black Cohosh – Lower back or neck tightness or pain; pelvic issues.

Black Currant – Insomnia in times of identity shifts and crises.

Blackberry Lily – Infertility, endometriosis, uterine tumors, bladder infections, sexual imbalances, genital inflammations, genital rashes or lower back problems with prostate, headaches.

Blessed Thistle – Stress in the stomach area.

Blue Vervain – Stress-related symptoms; difficulty sleeping; nightmares; heartburn; inflamations; tightness in the upper back, shoulders, and upper body (e.g. neck tension, dizziness, TMJ, eye strain and problems, earaches, headaches, rashes on the face and scalp); weakness in the lower body, (e.g. sluggish kidneys or stones, weakness or pain in the knees or ankles).

Borage – Many stomach ailments, reflux.

Celandine – Diseases and imbalances of the throat, tongue, larynx, or jaw.

Comfrey – Assists in healing bones after fractures or dislocations; also after surgery.

Elecampagne – Complementary therapy for a number of breathing difficulties in both animals and humans, especially asthma.

Fraxinella – Congestions; prone to inflammations.

Golden Amaranthus – Weakened immune system, a number of non-serious health problems, immune system weakened through long-term use of drugs.

Gravel Root – Kidney pains, urinary tract or bladder cysts, kidney stones.

Habanero Pepper – Vertigo; symptoms in the lower part of the body (lower back, kidneys, intestines, pelvic area, poor circulation, weakness in legs or knees).

Hemp Agrimony – Fears of bodily functions.

Horseradish – General lack of vitality and vigor; poor circulation; slow digestion or colds related to feelings of powerlessness and stagnation.

Hyssop – Stomach problems; problems, in general, of food assimilation and mineral deficiencies.

Lady's Mantle – Feeling of weakness, poor muscle tone, slumping posture, anemia, pale complexion.

Lemon Balm – Insomnia; stomach problems; headaches; tense muscles.

Lilac – Back and shoulder problems; poor posture.

Lobelia – Throat-centered imbalances; thyroid problems.

Lungwort – Lung problems, shallow or shortness of breath, addiction to tobacco, headaches, heart problems, stomach problems, ulcers.

Marshmallow – Heart problems, hardened arteries, hardened tissues.

Milk Thistle – Elevated liver enzymes, gall bladder problems, high blood pressure or heart problems.

Missouri Primrose – Eating disorders.

Motherwort – Endometriosis, bladder infections, sinus problems; symptoms related to early menopause.

Onion – Somatic symptoms from suppressed grief: including stomach and heart problems, as well as certain types of skin imbalances where there is a weeping rash or sores such as with puscular psoriasis. Also difficulty breathing, edema, susceptibility to colds.

Pink Lady's Slipper – Recurring headaches, sleeplessness, weaknesses in the legs, hips and lower organs.

Potato – Coldness in extremities.

Scarlet Pimpernel – Scalp or skin rashes.

Skullcap – Nervous tics.

Solomon's Seal – Muscular-skeletal/ligament tension and pain, such as problems with knees or joints.

Stinging Nettle – Addiction to drugs or alcohol.

Sumac – Long-term illnesses.

Teasel – Energy loss, aches, and pains due to such long-term illnesses as Lyme disease.

Water Lily – Symptoms involving the relation between heat and fluids: suceptabilty to infections, cysts, or boils; Heat or inflammations in the pelvic area: kidneys bladder, urinary tract, bowels, or prostate.

Wood Betony – Eating disorders, addictions.

PROTECTION (SEE ALSO "LOVE," "TRUST")

Golden Amaranthus – Connects us to the part of the self that "knows" that we are protected and guided on the highest level.

Hemp Agrimony – For many social fears. Opens one to understanding the interconnection of all life, and thereby enhances a feeling of safety.

Lady's Mantle – For those who feel unprotected, victimized, insecure, exposed. Protects the mental body from leakages from the emotions. Develops clarity.

Lemon Balm – Helps move tension and anxiety out; offers a calmness that provides protection against stress and breakdowns one can experience when overloaded.

Lovage – For moving into the world with a sense of safety and joy. Develops a sense of exhilaration and confidence in taking action.

Lobelia – Helps one feel safe in expressing feelings and opinions.

Motherwort – For those who feel vulnerable, threatened, used by others, unable say no. Balances inner softness with strength, assertiveness, setting healthy boundaries.

Pink Amaranthus – Helps a person who is feeling love to feel safe and protected.

Skullcap – For social difficulties and anxieties. Increases sense of safety, sense of self, and, consequently, increases ability to connect with others.

Teasel – For those who feel drained of energy. Protects one from energy leakage.

PRAYER – SEE "SPIRITUALITY"

PREJUDICE

Blackberry Lily – For those who have negative gender related attitudes. Releases sexual trauma and negative imprints.

Black Cohosh – For those who are prejudice against strong personalities.

Hemp Agrimony – For those who are judgmental or mistrustful; for feelings of alienation. Helps one access and develop the ability to connect to others.

Indian tobacco – For prejudice against certain types of religion or spiritual thought.

Jack-in-the-Pulpit – For prejudice against organized religion.

Marshmallow – For those who are intolerant, prejudiced, narrow-minded, inflexible. Strengthens one's ability to receive impulses from the heart and choose higher emotional values.

Motherwort – For those who are judgmental or prejudiced. Balances inner softness with strength, assertiveness and setting healthy boundaries.

Skullcap – For those who feel prejudice, antisocial, or judgmental. Allows the soul's natural sensitivities to the self and to others to open, both for specific short-term purposes, and as part of a longer-term therapeutic process.

PRIDE

Blue Vervain – For those who cannot yield to a safer, healthier, more practical approach because of their own pride, ambition, or role identity. Develops ease and versatility.

Marshmallow – For those who develop grudges because of pride. Helps soften the entire emotional system so that emotions are accessed, expressed, released, and forgotten in a shorter period of time.

Missouri Primrose – For those who cannot feel a healthy pride in themselves or their accomplishments. Helps one learn to accept and receive love, pleasure, and other forms of self-nurturing.

Solomon's Seal – For those who are not willing to change. Eases and softens extreme pride, arrogance, or willfulness. Helps one develop alternatives.

POWER

Blue Vervain – For those who feel obliged to live their lives in powerful roles. Balances the driven personality. Develops ease and versatility.

Borage – For discouragement. Strengthens a feeling of solidity, enhancing incarnation while individuality and commitment are renewed. Develops empowerment and goal-directed behavior, which, in turn, become part of the antidote for the state of defeat, helplessness, and powerlessness.

Golden Amaranthus – For a lack of ease or frustration even when one is very successful. Offers awareness of the power of the higher self and tuning into the ease of life.

Horseradish – For those who feel powerless. Old recurring thoughts or ideas receive energy to come forward for action or release; one feels more power/energy to act.

Lovage – For feeling the power of walking one's path.

Pink Lady's Slipper – For gentle souls, including artistic, mathematical, technological, altruistic or spiritually minded people. Helps one realize the beauty of one's being. Supports and strengthens those who embody this special kind of subtle or less overt power.

Wood Betony – For those who feel powerless to change or control behaviors. Stimulates higher reasoning, enabling one to act more in line with one's self concept.

PSYCHOTHERAPY – SEE "THERAPY"

PURIFICATION – SEE "RELEASE"

RELATIONSHIPS / FRIENDSHIPS

Black Cohosh – For those who attract dark or violent personalities unconsciously. Eases fear of violence, strong personalities, and of being hurt.

Black Currant – For those who have trouble ending relationships or moving on to new phases in their lives; for feeling slighted or ignored easily. Eases fears of abandonment and develops the courage to end the old and accept the new.

Blackberry Lily – For those who relive old patterns in new relationships; for fear of closeness and/or relationships; for those who feel victimized or betrayed by partners and friends.

Butterfly Weed – For inability to commit to long-term relationships; for the fear and sadness when the initial stages of "being in love" shift. Eases these fears allowing for more maturity and deeper relationship.

Celandine – For any breakdown in communication within a relationship or group. Enhances a sensitivity to feelings, intentions and orientations of others.

Elecampagne – For those who feel uncomfortable in social situations; for those who feel odd or different from others. Helps one feel comfortable with one's own uniqueness, easing much social turmoil and helping to connect with others.

Golden Amaranthus – For over-reliance on self, mistrustful of and frustration with others. Helps one to relax and to let down one's guard. Develops ease with people and life.

Indian Pipe – For those who are in non-loving relationships. Offers awareness of the presence of love.

Gravel Root – Helps those who suffer from loneliness or fear of being alone. Eases anxiety over friendships and relationships. Helps one gradually accept and benefit from periods of solace.

Hemp Agrimony – For many social and relationship fears. Helps access and develop the ability to connect to others. Feelings and perceptions of aloneness or disconnectedness are eased.

Marshmallow – For those who resolve relationship issues by ending them; for those who hold grudges, refuse to listen or won't compromise. Softens the entire emotional system so that emotions are accessed and released.

Motherwort – For many phases of conflict resolution, especially in couples therapy; for trouble in relationships; social fears; for those who feel vulnerable, threatened, used by others, or unable say no. Balances inner softness with strength, assertiveness, and setting healthy boundaries.

Stinging Nettle – Helps one become more aware of the basis of irrational responses and begin working with the deeper personal issues rather that degenerating to externalizing and blaming. Helps to heal deep hurts.

Pink Amaranthus – For numerous difficulties related to relationships; for those who unconsciously have attitudes that prevent relationships from developing in a healthy way. Helps one be reflective and heal some of the deeper issues of past relationships.

Skullcap – For social anxiety; for those at odds with friends. Allows the soul's natural sensitivities to the self and to others to open. For therapists who have personality differences with some clients.

Teasel – For conflicts in relationships; for relationship counseling. Helps couples discover how to balance the flow of energy between them so that one individual is not feeling used or taken advantage of.

Water Lily – For a needy personality; for those who scheme, control or manipulate. Helps one to receive unconditional affection and attention. Offers a sense of self-sufficiency and fulfillment.

White Columbine – For those searching for the "right" relationship. Provides a reassurance that "all is well" and unfolding in life. Eases feelings of inferiority, insecurity, and confusion.

Wood Betony – For those who prefer to be alone but are working on authentic ways to connect with others. Helps clarify deeper meanings of relationship, friendship, and sexuality.

Wormwood – For those who can't end a relationship, can't stop thinking about or are bothered by feelings towards another long after a relationship has ended. Releases and removes unconscious imprints.

RELAXATION – SEE "EASE OF LIFE"

RELEASE / REPRESSION

Note: "Release/ Repression" essences can bring suppressed and difficult emotions to the surface of consciousness, enabling them to be recognized and removed from the body-system. These essences are not recommended during pregnancy.

Blackberry Lily – For unconscious or unresolved problems in the past concerning close relationships. Heals deep fears around sexuality. Releases repressed sexual trauma.

Canada Thistle – For letting go of pain, guilt, or trauma that has been group or family inflicted.

Bull Thistle – For release of fears of being trapped, controlled, or confined.

Comfrey – Brings forward repressed parts of the self. Feelings, memories, and parts of the physical that may be shut down by the subconscious are opened.

Fraxinella – For creating movement or dealing with buried issues; for completion, purification, insight; for endings and beginnings; for release in final stages of healing trauma or for healing recent trauma. Helps with lingering confusion or pain.

Habanero Pepper – For stimulating the movement of repressed feelings while holding one in connection to the physical. Prevents separation and drifting; promotes clarity and presence.

Hemp Agrimony – For those who have a fear, memory, or feeling that it is unsafe to be with others, and so have many social fears. Assists in the release of such imprints.

Horseradish – Old recurring thoughts or ideas receive energy to come forward for action, release or manifestation. One feels more power/energy to act; obsessive thinking patterns are discarded.

Hyssop – For releasing guilt; helps those who have built personalities and lifestyles around guilt imprints; reawakens impulses of worthiness and receiving.

Indian Tobacco – For releasing subconscious fears or confusions around spiritual experiences or ideas, often bringing to the conscious mind information related to its origin, and so allowing fears to be more manageable. An even, stable reassurance and courage related to spirituality is brought into one's being.

Lungwort – Helps strengthen the lungs as a vehicle to release trauma, tension, and deep feelings, and to bring life-energy into the system.

Milk Thistle – For releasing deep anger, resentment, or other held feelings that block the flow of love. Allows forgiveness to lead to a deeper experience of love.

Onion – For releasing sadness. Helps all phases and aspects of the grieving process.

Scarlet Pimpernel – Helps with many aspects of difficult emotions. Can help one understand and transform intense emotions. Helps release of blocked energy in the heart. Treats obsession, anxiety, and fear.

Stinging Nettle – For releasing pain and grief related to partings and endings; for healing deep hurt from abandonment.

Wormwood – For those who feel stuck in old habits; for those who can't end a relationship; for release of unconscious imprints.

RESENTMENT – SEE "ANGER"

Resignation – see "Hope," "Pessimism"

Responsibility

Blue Vervain – For those who are driven or over-responsible. Helps develop ease and flexibility.

Butterfly Weed – For fear of commitment and responsibility because one fears losing freedom. Eases these fears, allowing for more maturity and deeper relationships.

Bull Thistle – For fear of being controlled or confined. One accepts responsibility more easily.

Golden Amaranthus – For those who feel they need to "do it all themselves." Reawakens awareness that we are guided and protected, allowing one to relax and let go of over-control and responsibility.

Lilac – For the overly responsible, or those who seem to fear accepting responsibility. Helps develop a healthy balance between self reliance and reliance on others.

Resistance / Avoidance

Black Currant – For those who resist growth and development due to fear of losing their sense of self.

Blue Vervain – For those who resist rest and relaxation. A sense of ease develops.

Bull Thistle – For those who unduly resist authority. Discernment develops.

Butterfly Weed – For those who resist commitment. Strength and certainty develop.

Fraxinella – For those who resist dealing with pain or difficult issues. Clarity and strength develop.

Golden Amaranthus – For those who resist the flow of life, always doing things the hard way. A sense of letting go and moving with the flow develops.

Indian Tobacco – For resistance to spirituality or spiritual practices. Releases subconscious fears of spirituality.

Jack-in-the-pulpit – For those who resist dialogue about their beliefs. Strengthens relationship to the inner voice.

Lady's Mantle – For those who resist their own feminine natures. Clarity develops.

Lilac – For those who resist or refuse help from others. Helps develop a healthy balance between self-reliance and reliance on others.

Lovage – For those who resist taking action. Certainty develops.

Onion – For those who resist the grieving process or facing past experiences of grief.

Marshmallow – For those who resist emotions or socialization. Inner softness develops.

Missouri Primrose – For those who resist the experience of their own self-worth. Self-appreciation develops.

Potato – For the tendency to sublimate or romanticize painful experiences. Brings a sense of stability in the growth process by providing a deep reference point of self when new experiences pull one off center.

White Columbine – For those who resist their calling or vocation. A sense of ease and clarity develops.

RESIGNATION / FATALISM

Bluebell – For those who dwell in the negative. Provides access to more positive aspects of personality.

Borage – For fatalism, depression or melancholy. Brings relief and offers peace, lightness and courage.

Sumac – For those who feel like giving up. Gives a strength to continue.

ROMANTIC LOVE

Black Cohosh – For those who attract dark or violent personalities unconsciously. Provides clarity, lifting the spell and revealing people for what they are and not what they pretend to be.

Blackberry Lily – For those who relive old patterns in new relationships; for those who fear closeness and/or relationship; for those who feel victimized or betrayed by partners and friends. Releases sexual trauma and relationship imprints from the past.

Butterfly Weed – For "love addiction"; for fear and sadness when initial stages of "being in love" shift; for those who cannot commit to long-term relationships. Eases these fears, allowing for more maturity and deeper relationship.

Celandine – For any breakdown in communication. Enhances sensitivity to feelings, intentions, and orientations of others. Assists in couples counseling, conflict resolution, and general frustration in any situation where one is not grasping the lesson being presented.

Pink Amaranthus – For numerous difficulties related to relationships; for those who unconsciously have attitudes and reflexes that are essentially protective in nature, but prevent relationships from developing in a healthy way. Helps one feel safe and trust in love.

Stinging Nettle – For those who want to get into a relationship when alone, and want to be alone when in a relationship. Helps one become more aware of the basis of one's irrational responses and begin working with one's deeper personal issues.

Teasel – For conflicts in relationships and relationship counseling. Helps couples discover how to balance the flow of energy between them so that one individual is not feeling used or taken advantage of.

White Columbine – For those searching for the right relationship. Provides a reassurance that "all is well" and unfolding in life.

Wormwood – For attachment to relationships that are unhealthy. Releases and removes unconscious imprints.

Wood Betony – For those who prefer to be alone but are working on authentic ways to connect with others. Helps clarify deeper meanings of relationship, friendship, and sexuality.

SADNESS

Borage – For feelings of burden, depression, or melancholy, worry or sadness. Brings relief and imparts feelings of peace, lightness, and courage.

Butterfly Weed – For fear and sadness when the initial stages of "being in love" shift. Eases these fears, allowing for more maturity and deeper relationship.

Indian Pipe – For sadness due to the lack of warmth and love in one's environment and the world. Expands awareness of the presence of universal love in every moment.

Lemon Balm – Stimulates peace allowing access to sadness.

Onion – For grief and sadness. Helps one process, express, and release sadness.

Star Jasmine – For heavy feelings associated with sadness. Lightens ones mood; brings the joy of spirit closer to one's consciousness.

SAFETY – SEE "TRUST," "PROTECTION"

SCHOOL-RELATED CONCERNS – SEE "STUDY"

SELF-ESTEEM

Elecampagne – For low-self esteem and when new feelings, talents, insights are awakened. Helps one to identify more deeply with newly discovered power and beauty in one's self.

Horseradish – For feelings of powerlessness, inadequacy, and low self-esteem, especially when the idea of moving forward evokes a fear that results in inertia. Eases feelings of frustration and powerlessness, Develops confidence.

Hyssop – For those who have built their personalities and lifestyles around guilt imprints. Releases guilt; reawakens impulses of worthiness and receiving.

Indian Pipe – For those who feel unloved, or that they need more love in their lives. Develops a sensitivity and receptivity to the presence of universal love.

Lilac – For those who do not feel comfortable or worthy to receive assistance from others due to either low self-esteem or very high standards; for those who set standards too high and thus create for themselves a cycle of lessening self-esteem through failure. Balances the relationship between self-reliance and reliance on others.

Missouri Primrose – For many aspects of low self-esteem; for those who cannot recognize or utilize their own power or value. Helps one learn to accept and receive love, friendship, goodness, pleasure, and other forms of energy that comfort and nurture the self.

Pink Lady's Slipper – For those who feel like they don't fit in. Helps one realize the unique beauty of one's being.

Skullcap – For those who can't accept themselves or who feel hatred towards themselves; for those who show signs of self-neglect. Allows the soul's natural sensitivities to the self and to others to open.

Stinging Nettle – For damaged or low self-esteem related to childhood pain. Accelerates associations made between early childhood pain and present stresses and difficulties. Helps to heal deep hurts.

Water Lily – For a needy personality. Helps one learn to receive unconditional affection or attention. Offers a sense of self-sufficiency and fulfillment.

White Columbine – For low self-esteem; for those who feel uncertain or confused in life choices. Provides a reassurance that "all is well" and unfolding in life.

Wood Betony – For those who judge or condemn themselves or feel unable to change or control their behavior. One feels less trapped by desires that do not align with one's self-concept.

Wormwood – For negative identities based on woundedness. Releases, breaks, and removes unconscious imprints.

SELF–EXPRESSION

Black Currant – For those who feel invisible; for fears that arise as identity and ideas of the self change. Offers the courage and illumination needed to look at and integrate new experiences and meanings of "self."

Celandine – Enhances all forms of expression.

Elecampagne – For balancing and integrating new identities. Develops ability to express one's uniqueness or newfound feelings, ideas and talents.

Horseradish – For feelings of powerlessness, and inability to manifest what one wants in life. Old recurring thoughts or ideas receive energy to come forward for action. Eases feelings of frustration and powerlessness, and enhances confidence.

Hyssop – For those who feel fear when successful or engage in self-sabotage. Releases guilt and shame imprints, adding clarity to self expression.

Jack-in-the-pulpit – For difficulties and conflicts expressing what one feels to be true. Strengthens the relationship to one's inner voice. Develops security and confidence in one's experiences, and the ability to give expression to them.

Lady's Mantle – For those who feel unexpressed. Enhances expression of creativity or spiritual development. Supports the expression of the feminine energies such as empathy, creativity, intuition, wisdom and spirituality, both for men and women.

Lovage – For moving into the world with a sense of safety and joy. Developing a sense of confidence and exhilaration in taking action.

Lobelia – For shyness or shame around expressing one's truth or sexuality. Offers courage to express, own and speak the truth regarding one's self.

Missouri Primrose – For those who are shy or inexpressive of their own truths. Enhances self-esteem and one's ability to self-nurture, thereby supporting one's self-expression.

Marshmallow – For those who are hurt, angry, or "hard" in their interactions with others. Helps social self-expression.

Pink Lady's Slipper – For those who have low self-esteem; for gifted people who have trouble fitting in or expressing the awareness they hold within. Helps one realize the beauty and subtle power of one's being, making it more available to the conscious mind for expression.

Skullcap – For those out of touch with themselves and others. Allows the soul's natural sensitivities to the self and to others to open. Gives one the ability to improve self-esteem and expression.

White Columbine – For those who feel lost or uncertain about their life purpose. Feelings of inferiority, insecurity, and confusion yield to a quiet strength and acceptance. Helps one find expression of self in career or vocation.

Wood Betony – For those who feel unexpressed. Stimulates a feeling of clarity regarding the self and its expression in the world.

SELF-SABOTAGE – SEE "SELF-EXPRESSION," "SHAME"

SENSITIVITY

Celandine – For communication blocks and misunderstandings. Enhances many aspects of communication and self–expression. Enhances inspiration or higher thought.

Indian Pipe – For stages when one is unaware of the presence of Love. Develops a sensitivity and receptivity to a higher love vibration; seeing and feeling the love in every moment.

Indian Tobacco – For insensitivity about spirituality that has its origin in deeper fears.

Jack-in-the-pulpit – For conflicts with or inability to resolve differences one feels between inner feelings and religious beliefs. Strengthens one's sensitivity to one's inner voice.

Japanese Knotweed – For group experience and ceremony. Enhances group awareness, sensitivity and telepathy.

Lobelia –For those confused, unclear, or not in touch with their feelings. Helps re-sensitize one to feelings or other realities that may have been lost.

Lady's Mantle – For those insensitive or unemotional. Enhances one's empathy and ability to feel. Imparts a feeling of strength and protection.

Marshmallow – For insensitivity to others in social situations. Softens the emotional body and increases sensitivity.

Potato – For the intellectually or spiritually minded who are insensitive to more mundane matters. Brings one more into the present and into the body, where one becomes aware of one's physical and emotional issues.

Skullcap – For numbness to others and life events; for those insensitive to or at odds with people. Allows the soul's natural sensitivities to the self and to others to open.

SEXUALITY

Blackberry Lily – For unconscious/unresolved problems in the past concerning close relationships; for deep fears around sexuality. Releases repressed sexual trauma.

Butterfly Weed – For obsessive sexual fantasies, for sexual addictions. Helps one develop a balance between love and freedom, and a more mature and deeper relationship.

Habanero Pepper – For sexual difficulties related to childhood trauma. Provides stability and connection to the physical as repressed trauma is moved to the surface.

Lobelia – For shyness or shame around expressing one's sexual nature. Develops courage to express, own, and speak the truth regarding one's self.

Pink Lady's Slipper – For problems with sexuality. Helps one realize the beauty of one's nature.

Star Jasmine – For those with a base or solely physical approach to sexuality. Uplifts or adds a spiritual perspective. Sexuality becomes more integrated with higher ideals; emotions become more aligned with spirituality; love becomes more unconditional.

Wood Betony – For resolving sexuality issues of individuals and couples. Stimulates a feeling of clarity regarding the self and its expression in the world.

SHAME

Blackberry Lily – For sexual shame. Releases sexual trauma and negative sexual imprints.

Hyssop – For shame, guilt, and self-sabotage,. Helps to cleanse the imprints of guilt, shame, and unworthiness, which prevent the person from accepting enjoyment and pleasure.

Jack-in-the-pulpit – For self-judgment, or feeling judged or misunderstood by a spiritual or religious community. Strengthens the relationship to one's inner voice, engendering a feeling of safety and confidence in one's inner experience. Helps in the expressing of new ideas and one's feelings.

Wood Betony – For shame or self-judgments around feeling unable to change. Eases struggle by stimulating higher brain functioning. One feels less trapped and controlled by desires that do not align with one's self-concept.

SHYNESS – SEE "SOCIALNESS / ANTI–SOCIALNESS"

SLEEP

Black Cohosh – For sleep disturbances resulting from fears of being hurt by others or obsessing about a personal relationship. For dreams of being trapped; for dreams of being pursued by vague dark forces.

Black Currant – For sleep disturbances resulting from fears of dying, or from fears when one's ideas of self or reality are challenged.

Blue Vervain – For difficulty sleeping, due to over-thinking, or when one is too wound up to relax; for nightmares and stress-related symptoms.

Bull Thistle – For sleep disturbances resulting from feeling confined, trapped, restrained, or suffocated.

Golden Amaranthus – For those who are tired but can't rest, or are have difficulty sleeping. Offers the awareness that we are protected and guided on the highest level, which allows one to relax and have restful sleep.

Indian Tobacco – For sleep disturbances from fears related to feeling the presence of dark forces.

Lemon Balm – For insomnia, inability to relax or fears related to resting. Provides a natural and deep relaxation, by easing the velocity of the mind, which can be agitated by fears that reside in the subconscious.

SLUGGISHNESS – SEE "STIMULATION"

SOCIAL ACTION – SEE "PEACE / PEACE-MAKING"

Socialness / AntiSocialness

Black Cohosh – For timidity and fear of confrontations. Helps one to remain engaged in dialogue, conflict, or negotiation without a reflex to avoid or disengage from the situation.

Celandine – For shyness, avoidance of socializing, difficulty speaking to others, feeling unexpressed or misunderstood. Enhances all aspects of self-expression and ability to understand others.

Elecampagne – For those who feel socially timid, shy, or rebellious; for those at odds or different from others or uncomfortable in social situations. Aids one in being comfortable with one's own uniqueness, easing much social turmoil by developing the ability to connect with others.

Hemp Agrimony – For many social fears; for feelings of disconnection and alienation. Helps one access and develop the ability to connect to others.

Indian Pipe – For those who feel unloved, lonely, frustrated and disappointed by relationships. Expands awareness of the presence of universal love.

Jack-in-the-pulpit – For those who feel inauthentic in their social or spiritual expression. Strengthens one's relationship to one's inner voice. Develops security, confidence and the desire to express one's experience.

Japanese Knotweed – For the development of group awareness, sensitivity and telepathy. Enhances group experience and ceremony.

Marshmallow – For antisocial behavior and hard-heartedness. Teaches one to feel social ease, and softens interactions.

Missouri Primrose – For those who are shy or unnexpressive. Develops self-esteem. Imparts an increased sense of safety and sense of self, and consequently increases one's ability to connect with others.

Skullcap – For those who feel the need to be alone; for social anxieties and insensitivities. Allows the soul's natural sensitivities to the self and to others to open.

Teasel – For those who over-give in relationships. Helps one learn to use energy in a balanced and judicious manner.

Speaking – see "Communication"

Spirituality (Prayer / Meditation)

Black Currant – For those who react to a profound spiritual experience – especially one that challenges previous beliefs – by escaping into subconscious denial; for questions about life and death that are no longer culturally or simplistically explained; for those who secretly deny metaphysical realities.

Blessed Thistle – For many stages of spiritual development; for clergy with doubts; for atheists with mental blocks; for the materialist closed to other possibilities of satisfaction. Helps one resume the soul's journey to the Divine by easing many of the fears and doubts that have been taught or developed regarding God's relationship to the human race and the individual.

Celandine – For those who feel frustrated or cut off from spiritual communication and connection in prayer or in communing with higher beings. Adds clarity to intuitive information one is receiving. Helpful when learning to connect with spirit guides, nature spirits, or angels.

Elecampagne – For times when new feelings and insights are awakened. Balances and integrates new experiences of spirituality.

Golden Amaranthus – For those who fear fate and sometimes spirituality. Helps awaken or open one's relationship with God or the Divine.

Hemp Agrimony – For disconnectedness, alienation, difficulty feeling "at home" in the world. Opens one to an aspect of love where one becomes aware of the interconnectedness of all things through the heart.

Hyssop – For those who have associated guilt with spirituality. Reawakens impulses of worthiness and receiving.

Indian Pipe – For those who can't feel God's presence or love; for those who feel deeply saddened or depressed by the absence of love and warmth in their environment and world. Develops sensitivity, receptivity, and awareness to the presence of Universal Love.

Indian Tobacco – For those who resist or avoid spirituality or spiritual practices. Helps to steady irrational fears or confusions. Releases subconscious fears of spirituality. Also for those who are genuinely seeking authentic spirituality. For those who have had a real spiritual experience and are confused by it. Keeps balance in the mental body during expanded states.

Jack-in-the-Pulpit – For aspects of developing one's personal and authentic spirituality. Helps one resolve conflicts between past spiritual experiences and present spiritual insight. Strengthens one's relationship to one's inner voice, enabling expression of authentic spirituality.

Japanese Knotweed – For enhancing group experience, ceremony, and ritual.

Lungwort For those practicing breathing meditation, yoga, kundalini, breathwork, or rebirthing. Helps bring life-energy into one's system.

Pink Lady's Slipper – For those who feel a special spiritual calling. Supports and strengthens those whose identity embodies subtlety and gentleness.

Potato – For those who, in seeking a spiritual life, are attracted exclusively to people, places, and things that produce a "high." Helps ground and integrate spiritual impulses or truths into the whole psyche. Also for stabilizing one's spiritual development so that it continues at an uninterrupted pace. Provides a foundation for balanced spiritual growth, and can be useful for many who have genuine spiritual experiences.

Star Jasmine – For the agnostic, materialistic, narrow-minded, or uninspired. Uplifts or adds a spiritual perspective. Increases insight and illumination in areas where the intellect receives inspiration from intuition.

Teasel – For energy loss due to an unbalanced spiritual or psychic experience. Restores and rebalances one's energy and auric field.

White Columbine – For those exploring the possibility of a more spiritual "vocation." Provides insight into true identity and highest purpose.

STAGNATION

Borage – For discouragement related to boredom or repetition or doing what one does not like to do. For those who feel stuck or afraid to make changes. Stimulates courage to face challenges and have hope.

Comfrey – For those who feel stuck in the therapeutic process. Helps one to access repressed memories and feelings.

Fraxinella – For those who feel that they cannot get past or resolve a personal, relationship or group issue. Releases frustration.

Habanero Pepper – Provides movement to repressed feelings, promoting clarity and presence. Holds one in connection to the physical while doing emotional work.

Horseradish – For feeling stuck in a feeling of powerlessness; for inability to change or have the life one wants. One feels more power and energy to act.

Lilac – Helps a general attitude of apparent "laziness," especially when a fear of lack of confidence causes this. Balances self-reliance and reliance on others.

Lovage – For difficulty manifesting plans into action, procrastination. Develops a sense of safety, joy, and exhilaration in moving into the world, and a confidence in taking action.

Lungwort – For working through emotional blocks between the solar plexus and jaw.

Milk Thistle – For those who are stuck in recurring patterns of suppression and episodes of anger. Helps one access repressed feelings and let go of old anger.

Scarlet Pimpernel – Stimulates movement of old, buried trauma into the consciousness.

Wood Betony – For those who feel stuck. Helps one wishing to solve a problem or issue to have access to clearer aspects of thinking and awareness.

Wormwood – For those who feel stuck in old habits, caught in the past, addicted, or unable to enjoy the present. Releases unconscious imprints.

STIMULATION (SEE ALSO "STAGNATION")

Borage – Stimulates courage to face challenges.

Fraxinella – Stimulates conscious interface with one's trauma.

Habanero Pepper –Stimulates clarity, presence, and groundedness while at the same time providing movement to repressed feelings.

Horseradish – Stimulates willingness to accept one's power.

Lemon Balm – Produces calmness and peacefulness as emotions are stimulated.

Lilac – Stimulate the ability to ask for help when needed.

Lovage – Develops a sense of safety, confidence, and exhilaration in walking one's path in the world.

Milk Thistle – Stimulates processing of anger.

Scarlet Pimpernel – Stimulates movement of old buried trauma.

Wood Betony – Stimulates higher brain function and reasoning to guide the individual in a situation, providing the lower nature more opportunity to evolve.

STRENGTH

Black Cohosh – For feeling strong in the face of conflict or interactions with diffi-cult personalities.

Borage – Imparts strength and courage.

Golden Amaranthus Feeling strength that allows letting go.

Horseradish – Helps one feel personal strength to undertake challenging tasks.

Lady's Mantle – For feeling strength and protection that supports the ability to contain and to use one's own feminine power.

Lovage – Imparts strength and joy.

Motherwort – Balancing inner softness with strength, assertiveness, and setting healthy boundaries.

Sumac – Imparts a strength to continue when faltering or giving up.

Teasel – For those who feel tired, weak, depleted, or emotionally exhausted. Helps one learn to use energy in a balanced and judicious manner. Rebalances loss of strength due to emotional conflicts.

STRESS

Black Currant – For the stresses that accompany deep work in the psyche, espe-cially when real change occurs.

Black Cohosh – For interpersonal stresses related to confrontation or interaction with strong personalities.

Blue Vervain – For mental stress; for those who try or work too hard. Ease and versatility develop.

Celandine – For stresses related to teaching, training, communication, under-standing. Enhance one's ability to communicate and understand others.

Golden Amaranthus – For the stress of feeling responsible; the stress of leader-ship. Eases the stress of daily performance and success, and helps one to relax and let go of over-control.

Gravel Root – For stresses related to aloneness. Enhances the ability to venture out on one's own and find solace in periods alone.

Lemon Balm – For mental turbulence; difficulty relaxing, anxiety, feeling over-loaded. Helps move tension and anxiety out. Imparts a calmness that provides a protection against stress and breakdowns.

Lobelia – For stresses related to self-expression and to difficulty in speaking.

Lungwort – For stresses that prevent proper breathing. Helps strengthen the lungs as a vehicle to release tension and deep feelings.

Marshmallow – For those who respond to stress by becoming tough or hard. For social stresses. Strengthens one's ability to receive impulses from the heart.

Water Lily – For stresses related to a need for attention.

Wormwood – Helps release stress held deeply in one's system.

STRUGGLE – SEE "EASE OF LIFE"

STUBBORNNESS – SEE "WILLFULNESS"

STUDY / SCHOOLWORK

Borage – For those who become discouraged and bored with school.

Blue Vervain – For those who stubbornly work until they collapse.

Celandine – For stubborn students who refuse to learn; for teachers, lecturers, students, and apprentices of any discipline. Enhances sensitivity to reception and transmission of information.

Comfrey – Helps with the retention of information after study.

Elecampagne – For those unwilling to learn and accept new ideas about themselves.

Golden Amaranthus – For those who stubbornly work against the tide. Helps one relax and go with the flow.

Habanero Pepper – For the alleviation of numerous forms of mental fogginess.

Japanese Knotweed – For general classroom ease.

Lilac – For those who stubbornly refuse help from others.

Pink Lady's Slipper – For those who are not challenged by school or do not fit in; for those who belong in a specialized learning environment.

Potato – For those who are very intellectually inclined and less "in touch" with daily matters.

Solomon's Seal – For those who resist change; for those who experience undue stress when plans change or things go wrong.

Star Jasmine – For those who cannot think clearly. Adds clarity to intellectual pursuits and increases insight and illumination to areas where the intellect receives inspiration from the intuition.

SUB–CONSCIOUS MEMORIES/EMOTIONS – SEE "REPRESSION"

SUBLIMATION – SEE "RESISTANCE"

TALKATIVE – SEE "SPEAKING"

TENSION – SEE "STRESS"

TIMIDITY – SEE "SOCIAL-NESS / ANTI-SOCIAL-NESS"

STRUGGLE – SEE "EASE OF LIFE"

STUBBORNNESS – SEE "WILLFULNESS"

STUDY / SCHOOLWORK

Blue Vervain – For those who stubbornly work until they collapse. Balance and better self-care develop.

Celandine – For all aspects of teaching and learning. Enhances sensitivity to information, reception and transmission of information.

Elecampagne – For those unwilling to accept new ideas about themselves, such as when learning new skills makes no impression on their self-concept. Helps one transition into a new identity, leaving older, negative imprints behind.

Golden Amaranthus – For those who stubbornly work against the tide. Helps one relax and go with the flow.

Habanero Pepper – For the alleviation of numerous forms of mental fogginess.

Lilac – For those who have difficulty learning to accept help from others.

Motherwort – For those who have difficulty learning to defend themselves.

Potato – For those who are very intellectual, and less "in touch" with ordinary matters. Brings one more into the present and into the body, where one becomes aware of one's physical and emotional issues. For who have flashes of genius. Provides a foundation for balanced mental growth.

Solomon's Seal – For those who resist change; for those who experience undue stress when plans change or things go wrong.

Star Jasmine – Adds clarity to intellectual pursuits and increases insight and illumination to areas where the intellect receives inspiration from the intuition.

SUB-CONSCIOUS MEMORIES/EMOTIONS – SEE "REPRESSION"

SUBLIMATION – SEE "RESISTANCE"

TALKATIVE – SEE "SPEAKING"

TENSION – SEE "STRESS"

TIMIDITY – SEE "SOCIALNESS / ANTISOCIALNESS"

THERAPY (INCLUDING PSYCHOTHERAPY, COUNSELING AND OTHER COMPLEMENTARY THERAPIES)

Blackberry Lily – For treating sexual trauma. Helps bring sexual trauma forward to the conscious mind. Good for therapy when one or both partners have had sexual trauma in the past.

Black Currant – For fears or resistance to therapy when change threatens the old identity.

Butterfly Weed – For treating love-addiction, promiscuity, or inability to commit to a relationship. Eases fears of being hurt or of being trapped, allowing for more mature and deeper relationships.

Bull Thistle – For treating claustrophobia and other types of phobias or obsessions related to being controlled or confined. Assists one in releasing negative past experiences of structure or authority. Helpful in various stages of recovery from rape, torture, or imprisonment.

Canada Thistle – For individual therapy, family therapy, or psychodrama, when issues related to family pain and trauma are being processed.

Celandine – For therapists and healers of all types. Enhances both the clarity and depth of the communication process.

Comfrey – For clients who have reached a plateau in therapy. Helps client go deeper into the therapeutic process.

Fraxinella – For short-term psychotherapy of recent victims of violent crimes and other traumas. Keeps the energies of hurt and pain from receding into the subconscious.

Habanero Pepper – For cerebral, analytical, spacey or aloof individuals who fear going into painful aspects of their personality during therapy.

Horseradish – For treatment of feelings of powerlessness or victimization.

Indian Tobacco – For those who fear the therapeutic process or certain types of therapists, therapy or healing.

Japanese Knotweed – For family or group therapy. Harmonizing of group energy, producing a sympathetic bond among all members.

Lady's Mantle – Instills mental and emotional clarity into the therapeutic process.

Lobelia – For those who cannot relate to or express certain or deeper aspects of themselves. For therapy related to sexuality or sexual identity.

Marshmallow – For clients who are cynical, opinionated, analytical, or angry, and who resist emotions. Softens the emotional body.

Milk Thistle – For treatment of suppressed anger or resistance to forgiveness.

Missouri Primrose – For treatment of unworthiness, poor self-esteem or inability to take care of one's self.

Motherwort – For clients who have difficulty setting boundaries; for many phases of conflict resolution, especially in therapy for couples.

Onion – For all stages of grieving; for bereavement counseling.

Potato – For use after any deep healing experience. Gently brings one back into "normal reality," where one can reflect on and integrate the experience.

Scullcap – Helps therapists develop empathy with those who are unlike them. A complement to Post Traumatic Stress Therapy (PTST) when one has retreated inwardly following a shock or trauma. Helps with rehabilitation in prison reform.

Star Jasmine – For psychotherapists and those who work directly with observable dysfunction, who may occasionally feel depressed, overwhelmed, or even fatalistic from having such close and regular association with these energies.

Solomon's Seal – Supportive in Post Traumatic Stress Therapy. Helps one learn to refocus and integrate the traumatic experience rather than react with anger and frustration.

Stinging Nettle – For individual, couple or family therapy when one who was traumatized as a child has reached adulthood and is re-exploring early family dysfunction. Accelerates associations made between early childhood pain and present stresses and difficulties.

Sumac – For those who have been in counseling for a long time. Helps renew the deeper motivation for the therapeutic process. Helps one feel the value of the work even when the impact might not be readily observable.

Teasel – For relationship counseling. Helps couples discover how to balance the flow of energy between them. Helps individuals who are feeling used or taken advantage of in relationship.

Wood Betony – For addiction treatment or any type of therapy involving behavior change or modification. Supports control of impulses.

Wormwood – For lingering negative or unwanted thoughts or feelings. Releases unconscious imprints. A useful complement to programs of behavior change.

THOUGHTS (UNWANTED, UNCLEAR) – SEE "CLARITY," "OBSESSIONS"

TRANSITION / TRANSFORMATION

Borage – For strength and courage in making transitions.

Black Currant – For those who hang on to old habits, have trouble ending relationships or moving on to new phases in their lives.

Golden Amaranthus – Eases transitions by helping develop a sense of ease and right direction. Helps those who struggle against life.

Jack-in-the-pulpit – Adds clarity to transitions that arise from one's true self. Strengthens one's relationship to one's inner voice.

Lady's Mantle – For mental and emotional clarity during transitions.

Lovage – For those who want to make changes in their lives or want to begin taking action on an idea or plan.

Scarlet Pimpernel – For many aspects of difficult emotions that are buried in the psyche and influence more conscious values and attitudes. Helps one understand, transform and release intense emotions.

Solomon's Seal – Softens extreme pride, arrogance, or willfulness; helps one develop alternatives.

Sumac – For those who feel feel like giving up. Assists in maintaining connection with the heart during difficult phases and transitions in recovery, brings strength and stamina to the individual.

TRAUMA

Black Cohosh – For treating early trauma from a strong, abusive personality. Helps those who fear confronting or dealing with strong personalities.

Blackberry Lily – For repressed sexual trauma. Helps bring the information needed forward to the conscious mind.

Bull Thistle – For treating trauma that causes fear of being trapped, controlled or confined.

Canada Thistle – For pain or trauma that has been group or family inflicted.

Fraxinella – For treating recent trauma or old, burried trauma that is beginning to surface.

Habanero Pepper – For separation or drifting while doing emotional work. Holds one in connection to the physical. Promotes clarity and presence, while at the same time moving repressed feelings related to trauma to the surface.

Lady's Mantle – Brings clarity to the individual when processing trauma.

Lemon Balm – For times when memories of trauma surface to the conscious mind. Produces a peace, calm and clarity that allows deeper exploration or work.

Lilac – For early trauma, causing a difficul burden for an individual; refusing help from others.

Lungwort – Helps strengthen the lungs as a vehicle to release trauma, tension, and deep feelings, and to bring life-energy into the system.

Scarlet Pimpernel – For buried trauma that is lodged in the system. Helps old pain to surface for releasing.

Solomon's Seal – Supportive in Post Traumatic Stress Therapy. Helps one learn to refocus and integrate the traumatic experience rather than react with anger and frustration.

Stinging Nettle – For treating trauma that distorts perception or skews emotions. For treating the pain and sadness of early family break-ups.

Teasel – For anger that is recent, intense, and drains energy suddenly and dramatically; for energy loss due to fighting and arguments. Helps to rebalance energy loss due to emotional trauma.

TRUST

Blessed Thistle – For those who have difficulty trusting the Divine. Helps ease one's fears, doubts, and misgivings regarding God's relationship to the human race and to the individual.

Golden Amaranthus – For those who have difficulty trusting the flow of life. Offers awareness of protection and guidance on the highest level, allowing one to let one's guard down, to trust, to enjoy, to go with the flow, to "let go and let God."

Hemp Agrimony – For those who are mistrustful, judgmental, on guard or reluctant to socialize; for feeling that it is unsafe to be with others.

Lilac – For those who burden themselves, refusing help from others. Helps in developing qualities of balanced self-reliance and trust.

UNCONSCIOUS MEMORIES/EMOTIONS – SEE "REPRESSION"

UNDERSTANDING – SEE "AWARENESS"

UNCERTAINTY – SEE "CERTAINTY"

UNWORTHINESS – SEE "SHAME," "SELF-ESTEEM"

VICTIMIZATION – SEE "PROTECTION"

VIOLENCE – SEE "ANGER," "TRAUMA"

VOCATION – SEE "WORK"

WEAKNESS – SEE "STRENGTH"

WILLFULNESS

Blue Vervain – For strong-willed people who overwork and neglect taking care of themselves. A sense of safety and versatility develops, easing the "overdrive" state.

Golden Amaranthus – For those who try again and again even when all outward signs say to stop or to try something else; for over-use of will forces that eventually can cause breakdowns in both health and relationships.

Solomon's Seal – For those who experience stress or extreme difficulty when things do not go as planned; for those who are not willing to change. Softens extreme willfulness, pride, arrogance; helps one develop alternatives.

Work / Vocation

Blue Vervain – For those who live their lives as leaders, role models, or providers; for strong-willed people who overwork and neglect taking care of themselves.

Borage – For discouragement related to boredom or repetition or doing what one does not like to do. Offers a feeling of presence, grounding, embodiment, even stoutheartedness.

Elecampagne – For those learning to identify more deeply with newly discovered gifts or talents. Integrates them into one's identity.

Golden Amaranthus – For those whose true identity and vocation are masked by tendencies to take on too much work or to take high risks. For those who are often charismatic and original and succeed through personal effort; yet, are willful, frustrated, perfectionist, and competitive, with swings of intense energy and depletion.

Jack-in-the-pulpit – For those working in or seeking a vocation within religious/spiritual groups. Provides a bridge between incoming spiritual impulses and one's day-to-day expression of spirituality in the world.

Japanese Knotweed – For group discord, lack of productivity in groups, lack of acceptance among group members; for those who are not team players. Harmonizes group energy, producing a sympathetic bond among all members.

Lady's Mantle – For those who feels uncertain about identity or career. Develops self-awareness and confidence.

Lovage – For those unable to enjoy work or frustrated about their life direction. Develops a sense of safety, joy, and exhilaration in walking one's path, and confidence in taking action. For those who are fearful, uncertain, or timid when taking action toward a new goal.

Lobelia – For uncertainty about one's ideas and opinions, and lack of clarity about goals. Offers the courage to express, own and speak the truth regarding one's own self.

Missouri Primrose – For those who work too much, postpone enjoyment, push themselves. Helps one accept and receive love, friendship, goodness, pleasure, and other forms of self-nurturing. Vital energies taken in through self-nurturing are converted into confidence and goal-directed activities.

Pink Lady's Slipper – For gifted people who have trouble fitting themselves into vocational choices. Supports and strengthens the awareness of their unusual talents.

Star Jasmine – For those who are looking for more inspiration in their problem-solving processes. Adds clarity to intellectual pursuits and increases insight and illumination to the areas where the intellect receives inspiration from intuition.

Sumac – For those who feel that they have somehow missed out in life or have been passed by. Sustains drive and energy as one works towards a long-term goal.

Teasel – For those whose work does not resonate with the soul, for those who seek "right livelihood."

White Columbine – For those who are uncertain or confused about life-direction, life-choices or vocation. Offers certainty and clarity on life-path.

WORTHINESS – SEE "SHAME"

WORRY

Black Cohosh – For those who worry about violence or being hurt by others.

Blessed Thistle – For those who worry about the future or the next disaster in their lives.

Blue Vervain – For worry due to high stress and feeling driven or obligated to be providers or leaders; for those who worry because of intense feelings of responsibility.

Borage – For worry, melancholy or sadness. Gives relief, peace, lightness and courage.

Black Currant – For those who worry about being abandoned or of not existing.

Bull Thistle – For those who worry about being trapped or confined.

Golden Amaranthus – For fretfulness or worry that comes about by feeling one must control one's fate; for those who worry about what might happen.

Gravel Root – For those who worry about being alone.

Hemp Agrimony – For those who worry in social situations.

Indian Tobacco – For worry about death or dying.

Lemon Balm – For those who are prone to worry or anxiety.

Lilac – For those who worry after delegating a task to another.

Lobelia – For those who worry about what they say.

Sumac – For those who worry that life is passing them by.

Wormwood – For obsessive, chronic or irrational worry about the past or old issues beyond one's control.

www.ingramcontent.com/pod-product-compliance
Lightning Source LLC
Chambersburg PA
CBHW080331270326
41927CB00014B/3177